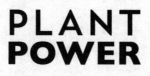

PLANT
POWER

PLANT POWER

Flip
Your Plate,
Change
Your Weight

IAN K. SMITH, M.D.

ST. MARTIN'S PRESS
NEW YORK

First published in the United States by St. Martin's Press, an imprint of St. Martin's Publishing Group

PLANT POWER. Copyright © 2022 by Ian K. Smith. All rights reserved. Printed in the United States of America. For information, address St. Martin's Publishing Group, 120 Broadway, New York, NY 10271.

www.stmartins.com

Library of Congress Cataloging-in-Publication Data

Names: Smith, Ian K., author.
Title: Plant power : flip your plate, change your weight / Ian K. Smith, M.D.
Description: First edition. | New York : St. Martin's Press, 2022. | Includes index.
Identifiers: LCCN 2021051057 | ISBN 9781250278029 (hardcover) | ISBN 9781250278036 (ebook)
Subjects: LCSH: Nutrition. | Natural foods. | Health.
Classification: LCC RA784 .S587 2022 | DDC 613.2—dc23/eng/20211122
LC record available at https://lccn.loc.gov/2021051057

Our books may be purchased in bulk for promotional, educational, or business use. Please contact your local bookseller or the Macmillan Corporate and Premium Sales Department at 1-800-221-7945, extension 5442, or by email at MacmillanSpecialMarkets@macmillan.com.

First Edition: 2022

10 9 8 7 6 5 4 3 2 1

To Tristé.

Absolutely always.

There's no doubt that you showed me the way!

XOXO

ACKNOWLEDGMENTS

I was at a charity golf tournament many years ago and met this guy who was extremely affable, chatty, and a good sport. We had a nice conversation as is typical at these celebrity affairs, and he gave me his card and told me if I ever needed anything to look him up. I looked down and saw that he was the COO of St. Martin's Press. I found this ironic as at the time I was being published at another major house.

A couple of years later, I had a book rejected by the house that had published the first of a two-book deal. I had nowhere to go, but I did have an idea for a diet book that came from my work on the TV show *Celebrity Fit Club*. Unfortunately, that too was politely turned down by a couple of major houses, and with no options left, I was in a bit of a quandary. I had spent all my advance money and royalties from previous books and my other income at the time was meager at best. My brother tried to convince me to self-publish the diet book that had been rejected. I hemmed and hawed as I thought it beneath me to self-publish versus being published by a major house. My brother—who can be very motivating and convincing—eventually won me over to his point of view and I published that book. It was called *The Fat Smash Diet*. I sold so many books off my website that it crashed within an hour of my appearance on *The View*. I simply could not

ACKNOWLEDGMENTS

handle the pace and volume of orders for this little book that had been rejected and constructed in my brother's small apparel design showroom in downtown New York City. Calling the book's production and finished product "rough" is being kind.

I then remembered that nice, affable guy I had met at the golf tournament. I found his card, called him, and told him I needed help. I needed a major publisher to take over the book and publish it the way big publishers do. He agreed, of course, to have me meet one of his high-octane editors and see if she was interested in buying the book and "republishing" it. I had only been selling the little book for a month. The editor met with me in the guy's office and, once hearing my sales numbers, agreed on the spot that she wanted it. St. Martins took the book and gave it some sheen and put it out on the market, and it instantly went to #1 on the *New York Times* bestseller list where it stayed for months.

That book changed my life, literally and figuratively. That kind, funny, chatty guy was absolutely instrumental in making that happen. He was an angel in a dark sky. I am forever indebted to him. He has since semiretired, but his impact on my life and career are still as poignant today as they were when I sat in his office looking for a lifeline. His name is Steve Cohen. I love him like a brother, even though he's a terrible golfer and I always take his money on the course. (Well, most of the time!)

CONTENTS

A NOTE FROM THE AUTHOR

This might be the most personal health book I've ever written. I have been a happy omnivore my entire life, enjoying my cabbage and sweet potatoes as much as I have my steak and juicy burgers. I love the taste and texture of meat, and the thought of never being able to eat my honey-glazed salmon or barbecued short ribs causes me to quiver. As I've gotten older, however, I have noticed that my body responds differently to a heavily animal-based meal. It seems to stick around in my digestive tract longer, and I feel more sluggish than I remember feeling when I was younger.

People close to me have been vegans, vegetarians, pescatarians, and almost any "-tarian" you can imagine, but I have happily and confidently continued on my path of eating whatever I want from both the plant and animal world, all in moderation. I was never one to have a steak for breakfast or a burger stacked so high I'd have to almost break my jaw hinge to open my mouth wide enough to eat it. I ate meat when I wanted, but I didn't crave it or feel unsatisfied if it wasn't on the dinner menu. Given that I've been a fitness enthusiast my entire life and continue to press a lot of iron in the gym, I also believed for a long time that I needed the meat protein to build and maintain bigger and stronger muscles. Then something happened. A news alert came across my phone, bringing my attention to an article about bodybuilders and endurance athletes who had given up red meat and had become plant-based eaters and saw no diminution in their muscle size or strength. In fact, they talked about their increased energy levels and feelings of wellness with their new style of eating.

I did what I always do when intrigued—I studied and learned and dug into the facts as well as experiential reporting of others. I realized that this plant-based eating was something I wanted to try. No more bacon every morning or steaks twice a week. I would slowly reduce my consumption of red meat, increase my intake of fruits and vegetables, and eat more lean chicken and fish when I had the urge. I must be honest and tell you that it was an adjustment at first. I found myself having to avoid the butcher section of the grocery store, which was always my second stop after the produce section. I started ordering my pancakes without bacon and opting for a chicken sandwich instead of the burger that seemed to be calling my name. I didn't tell anyone what I was doing; I just changed my eating habits quietly without fanfare, keeping a checklist in my mind of how many times I sat down to a meal that didn't have any red meat or poultry and feeling proud of myself when I could go an entire week without a steak or a burger.

The results were immediate. I felt lighter, more energetic, and more present. My weight lifting didn't suffer with this new dietary change, and I started trying new recipes and meal combinations that never caught my attention in the past, but I quickly learned what I had been missing all these years. I'm not a vegan or vegetarian, but I'm not the big meat eater that

I used to be either. I've found that eating more plant-based not only made me feel better but saved me a lot of money and gave me greater flexibility when eating out at different restaurants around the world. There's always something I can find on the menu since meat is no longer a requirement. You too can make this easy transition to plant-based eating and not only experience the truly transformative powers of plants but pitch in and help save the planet while doing so. *Plant Power* gives your life the proverbial efficiency of "two birds with one stone"—well, maybe two heads of cabbage instead!

Ian K. Smith, M.D.
April 2022

I

The LIFE-CHANGING
POWER
OF PLANTS

Let me start by saying that this is not a book that's trying to convince you to become a vegan or a vegetarian. I am neither, but I have absolutely no problem with people who decide that is how they want to eat and live. I like and eat all types of food, and I don't feel guilty for doing so. However, what I've learned over the years is that what I consume and the rates at which I consume certain foods, ingredients, and beverages is something that I should reconsider and be willing to reevaluate, as I believe our diets and how we treat our bodies should be in perpetual evolution. I have always understood and respected the power of plants, but I have been lagging in implementing more of their potential into my daily nutrition regimen—until now.

It really goes back to when we were children. At some point in our lives, we've all heard from a parent or a teacher, "Make sure you eat your fruits and vegetables." This instruction was more than just another developmental cliché; rather, it came from centuries of scientific research and observation that have for a long time explained the magical and impactful powers of plants on our entire bodies, including our minds and outlooks on life.

Simply put, plants help prevent and treat numerous illnesses, and they increase not only the length of our lives but the quality as well. People who eat more plant-based foods tend to have lower rates of obesity, heart disease, cholesterol levels, and cancer, among other things. Studies have also found that people who predominantly eat plant-based diets are more active, and their habitus tends to be leaner.

So what is it about plants that makes them so powerful? It's all built into their nutritional profile, which makes them without peer. When you do a side-by-side nutritional comparison of plant-based foods and animal-based foods, the numbers speak for themselves. Eating a predominantly plant-based diet means that you will consume more concentrated amounts of vitamins, minerals, and antioxidants (disease fighters that neutralize dangerous free-radical compounds). Plant-based foods also tend to be lower in the less healthy saturated fats and cholesterol, both of which can lead to heart and blood vessel disease and all the related medical complications that follow.

Why should you eat more plant-based foods? That answer is quite simple. They are overwhelmingly the best fuel for our bodies and help us both prevent and fight disease. Most early forms of medications came from plants by way of herbal remedies. Their medicinal properties have been known and used for thousands of years and are still used today around the world. Food should be fun and tasty and bring great pleasure, but it also should be considered for its quality to fuel our bodies so that we remain healthy, fight disease, and achieve peak performance in whatever we ask of ourselves, whether it be a physical or mental task.

The benefits of a plant-based diet have been well documented and universally accessible to those who desire and can afford to load up on these nutritional powerhouses. Thousands of studies have been conducted around the world looking at various aspects of plant-based diets and how they directly and indirectly impact the quality and length of our lives. Below you will find just a sampling of the benefits you can derive from loading up on the plants and keeping your animal product consumption to a much smaller fraction of your dietary regimen. Let's be clear—I love a juicy rib eye as much as anyone else, but studying and learning about all the wonderful health advantages I can get from eating more plant-based foods has inspired me not to give up my steaks but to increase the gaps between the times I eat them. While at first I thought it might be difficult, I've never felt stronger or more alive since I made the switch. The increased energy level I experienced is something that has been found in several studies, including one published in *Public Health Nutrition* in which researchers found a 50 percent decrease in the prevalence of hyperthyroidism (overactive thyroid) in those who largely consumed a plant-based diet compared to those who consumed an omnivorous diet (one in which plants and animal products are eaten).[1] Hyperthyroidism can cause decreased energy because it leads to increased metabolism that

---

1. Serena Tonstad et al., "Prevalence of Hyperthyroidism According to Type of Vegetarian Diet," *Public Health Nutrition* 18, no. 8 (2015): 1482–7, doi: 10.1017/S1368980014002183.

leads to exhaustion. It's akin to a battery-operated device constantly running without being charged. Eventually, the battery will run out of power, and the device will shut down.

BENEFITS OF A PLANT-BASED DIET

Lower your cholesterol

Reduce risk for heart disease

Lower your blood pressure

Help with weight loss

Reduce risk for cancer

Help you live longer

Reduce risk for stroke

Reduce risk for diabetes

Increase energy

Improve immune system function

Boost your mood

LOWER CHOLESTEROL

High levels of cholesterol in the blood can be very dangerous. Too much cholesterol can lead to fatty deposits that stick to the interior walls of our blood vessels, causing the opening through which blood flows to narrow. This narrowing causes the blood flow to be restricted or limited. Imagine taking a water hose and squeezing it from the outside. Water can still flow, but much less than before you applied the restrictive pressure. Reduced blood flow is not a good situation, because the body needs blood to circulate as fast and as full as it can to reach all our organs and tissues so they can be properly nourished with the nutrients being carried within the blood plasma. When blood vessel disease develops (this usually takes time and is typically a quiet process until enough damage has occurred to cause a problem), it can lead to all kinds of problems, including heart disease, heart attacks, kidney disease, eye disease, and strokes. Research has convincingly shown that transitioning from a predominantly animal-based diet to one that's plant-based can lower the LDL (bad) cholesterol by 10 to 15 percent and by as much as 25 percent for those who go strictly vegan.

FOODS AND NUTRIENTS THAT MAY HELP LOWER CHOLESTEROL

Avocados
Fiber (oats, beans, legumes, fruits, vegetables)
Fenugreek seeds and leaves
Liquid vegetable oils (canola, olive, sunflower, safflower)
Nuts (almonds and walnuts)
Red yeast rice
Soybeans (tofu and soy milk)
Whey protein
Yarrow plant (tea)

REDUCE HEART DISEASE RISK

Two big contributors among many when it comes to heart disease are excessive blood levels of cholesterol and saturated fats. Meat and other animal-based foods are high in both of these heart-unfriendly compounds, so replacing them with more plant-based foods can pay important health dividends. Many studies, including one by the American Heart Association, found that eating a plant-based diet reduced the risk of cardiovascular disease by 16 percent, and the risk of dying from the disease was reduced by approximately 31 percent. It's important to note that the type of plant-based foods also matters. Fruits, vegetables, healthy oils, whole grains, and legumes are where your efforts should be focused while avoiding unhealthy plant foods, such as refined grains (cookies, cakes, and doughnuts) and sugary beverages like soda and certain sweet teas that have little or no nutritional value at all. The American Heart Association gives guidelines on how we can eat better for our hearts.

HEART FOODS

EAT MORE

- Variety of fruits and vegetables
- Whole grains
- Nontropical vegetable oils (canola, corn, olive, peanut, safflower, soybean, sunflower, etc.)

- Nuts
- Legumes
- Low-fat dairy products
- Skinless poultry and fish

EAT LESS

- Saturated fat
- Trans fat (also called *hydrogenated oil* and *partially hydrogenated oil*)
- Sodium
- Red meat
- Sweets
- Beverages with added sugars (like soda and some iced teas)

LOWER YOUR BLOOD PRESSURE

High blood pressure (hypertension) is often called the "silent killer," because it can go undetected for years before the damage it does becomes evident and often leads to a catastrophic event like a stroke or a heart attack. Unfortunately, suffering from this condition for a length of time can lead to several medical complications, including heart disease, type 2 diabetes, and kidney failure. The good news is that multiple studies have shown that eating a plant-based diet can significantly lower blood pressure in many people, and one study showed that vegetarians had a 34 percent lower risk of developing hypertension compared to nonvegetarians.[2]

It's important that you check your blood pressure at least once or twice a year if you have no underlying medical conditions and haven't been diagnosed with high blood pressure. If you have received this diagnosis, then work with your healthcare provider to figure out a schedule of how many times it should be checked. It's also important that you know what is considered normal versus abnormal blood pressure. Use this table from the American Heart Association to help you make sense of your numbers.

BLOOD PRESSURE CATEGORY	SYSTOLIC mm Hg (upper number)		DIASTOLIC mm Hg (lower number)
Normal	Less than 120	and	Less than 80
Elevated	120–129	and	Less than 80
High Blood Pressure Stage 1	130–139	or	80–89
High Blood Pressure Stage 2	140 or higher	or	90 or higher
Hypertensive Crisis (immediately call your doctor or go to the emergency room)	Higher than 180	and/or	Higher than 120

---

2. Hao-Wen Liu et al., "Vegetarian Diet and Blood Pressure in a Hospital-Base Study," *Ci ji yi xue za zhi [Tzu-Chi Medical Journal]* 30, no. 3 (2018): 176–80, doi: 10.4103/tcmj.tcmj_91_17.

The good news about eating more plants is that extensive research has been conducted regarding plant-based diets and their impact on lowering blood pressure. There's evidence suggesting there's a connection, and researchers have even identified various foods that have a greater chance of delivering significant impact. Check them out below and load them up in your grocery cart.

BLOOD PRESSURE–LOWERING FOODS

Bananas	Leafy green vegetables
Beets	Lentils (and other legumes)
Blackberries	
Blueberries	Oats
Cinnamon	Olive oil
Dark chocolate	Pomegranates
Fermented foods (apple cider vinegar, kimchi, kombucha, miso, natural yogurt, tempeh)	Seeds (pumpkin, flax, sunflower)
	Tree nuts (especially pistachios)
Garlic	Watermelon
Kiwis	

LOSE WEIGHT

Many people who have made the switch from an animal-based diet to one that's plant-based have been rewarded with not only better health but also weight loss, even if that was not their original intention. There's no doubt that for most people who begin to eat predominantly plant-based meals, their risk of obesity decreases. A major study in *Diabetes Care* found there to be a substantial body mass index (BMI) difference between non–meat eaters and meat eaters.[3]

There are several reasons why many experience this weight-loss benefit when eating more plant-based foods. First, these foods tend to be lower in calories when compared to animal-based foods such as meat and dairy. The fewer calories you eat, the more likely you will lose weight or avoid putting on excess weight. Second, whole grains and vegetables typically have a lower glycemic index (GI), which means they are digested more slowly, thus leading to a slower, evener rise in blood sugars. Third, these foods tend to be much higher in fiber, and this is beneficial, because fiber gives us a longer feeling of fullness, which means we will be less hungry and eat less often.

There is one caveat that must be mentioned when it comes to the presumption that a plant-based diet automatically means someone is going to lose weight or get thinner. There are plenty of vegans and vegetarians who struggle with weight problems just the way people who consume animal-based diets do. It can be confusing when you associate diets full of meat and other animal-based products full of calories and compare them to plant-based foods, which you assume would be just the opposite. How does someone gain weight or not be able to lose weight when they're eating less of the "bad" stuff and more of

3. Serena Tonstad et al., "Type of Vegetarian Diet, Body Weight, and Prevalence of Type 2 Diabetes," *Diabetes Care* 32, no. 5 (2009): 791–6, doi: 10.2337/dc08–1886.

the "good" stuff? The answer is pretty simple. Depending on how and with what you cook and eat your plant-based foods, you can still load them with excess calories (butter, cream, heavy sauces, frying). Regardless of what type of food you eat, the fundamental rule still stands—consuming more calories than you burn will lead to weight gain, and that still holds even if you've been eating nothing but large kale salads and quinoa.

REDUCE CANCER RISK

Cancer is the second-leading cause of death in the U.S., and it's a complicated and frustrating disease process that not only afflicts millions of people each year but also baffles medical experts and researchers who constantly study its causes and ways to prevent and treat it. Often, it's difficult to point to one thing that actually triggers the cancer process, as there tend to be multiple factors involved (genes, environmental toxins, poisons, and other carcinogens). Nonetheless, research suggests a plant-based diet could help reduce one's cancer risk. Nutrients that help protect us against cancer include vitamins, minerals, fiber, and phytochemicals (plant chemicals). These nutrients can be found in large supply in beans, fruits, nuts, seeds, and vegetables.

Red meat has been heavily studied, and it's been found that the more we eat of it, the greater our risk of dying from all causes. When red meat is cooked, chemical compounds are created that are thought to contribute to the cancer development process. In fact, the International Agency for Research on Cancer (IARC) evaluated more than eight hundred studies looking at the association of cancer with eating processed red meat and unprocessed red meat and concluded that the risk of developing cancer rises with the amount consumed. Each 50-gram portion of processed meat (e.g., 3.5 slices of bacon) eaten daily increases the risk of colorectal cancer by 18 percent.[4] The IARC goes on to conclude that those who eat a predominantly plant-based diet along with a moderate amount of fish can experience a 45 percent reduced risk for colorectal cancers when compared to those whose diets include meat. If you're going to eat meat, make sure you consume a greater proportion that is unprocessed rather than processed.

KNOW YOUR MEATS

PROCESSED RED MEAT

Bacon

Beef jerky

Ham

Salami

Sausage

UNPROCESSED RED MEAT

All fresh and frozen cuts of beef, goat, lamb, pork, veal, and venison

---

4. Véronique Bouvard et al., "Carcinogenicity of Consumption of Red and Processed Meat," *Lancet Oncology* 16, no. 16 (2015): 1599–600, doi: 10.1016/S1470-2045(15)00444-1.

LOWER STROKE RISK

There are multiple factors that can increase your risk for stroke, including high blood pressure, smoking, diabetes, diets high in bad fats, physical inactivity, high cholesterol, obesity, coronary heart disease, carotid artery disease, peripheral artery disease, and sickle cell anemia. Many of these factors can be significantly reduced by following a plant-based diet and making healthier lifestyle choices. In fact, half of all strokes are preventable. The even better news is that research has shown that the highest consumers of fruits and vegetables have a 21 percent lower risk of stroke than those who consumed the least.[5]

LOWER DIABETES RISK

The relationship between our diets and type 2 diabetes has been long established. The more overweight and obese a person, the greater their risk for developing this condition in which the body is unable to adequately process the sugar that's floating in the blood. Being overweight typically means that we have more fat, and having more fat means the greater likelihood of our body developing insulin resistance, which means the body doesn't properly respond to the all-important insulin hormone that's critical in regulating blood sugar levels.

---

5. Dan Hu et al., "Fruits and Vegetables Consumption and Risk of Stroke: A Meta-Analysis of Prospective Cohort Studies," *Stroke* 45, no. 6 (2014): 1613–9. doi: 10.1161/STROKEAHA.114.004836.

Plant-based diets contribute to weight loss, which means a reduction in the amount of fat tissue we have in our bodies, and thus the less chance of our insulin hormone not working properly. One study found that eating a plant-based diet filled with high-quality plant foods was effective at reducing the risk of developing type 2 diabetes by a whopping 34 percent.

Diabetes can be a complicated disease; no two people have all the same triggers or respond the exact same way to treatment. Every diabetic needs to know what foods and treatments are best for managing their illness, but in many cases, weight loss and a diet low in processed sugars and high in fiber and plant-based whole grains can make a difference. Here are some foods that could be beneficial for the prevention and management of diabetes.

DIABETIC-FRIENDLY FOODS

Beans and other legumes

Fruit (fresh or frozen/canned without sugar)

Green leafy vegetables

Vegetables (raw, steamed, roasted, or grilled)

Walnuts

Whole grains (amaranth, brown rice, oatmeal, quinoa, etc.)

IMPROVE IMMUNE SYSTEM FUNCTION

The world's recent challenge with the COVID-19 pandemic taught us many things, especially the importance of a strong immune system. Plant-based eating is essential to making sure our immune systems are in their best shape. Plants that are full of vitamins, minerals, phytochemicals, and antioxidants help our cells stay healthy and maintain the proper biologic balances in our bodies so that our immune systems can function at peak performance. When germs and other microorganisms invade our bodies, we need an immune system that is prepared and strong enough to defend us from the dangers of infection. While there are lots of nutrients that can help bolster our immune systems, vitamins B, C, and D and zinc top the list. Below are some foods that contain immune-boosting nutrients.

IMMUNE-BOOSTING FOODS

Almonds

Broccoli

Citrus fruits

Garlic

Ginger

Green tea

Kiwis

Papayas

Red bell peppers

Shellfish (crab, lobster, mussels, oysters, shrimp)

Spinach

Sunflower seeds

Turmeric

Yogurt (brands that specifically contain probiotics and/or live cultures)

BOOST YOUR MOOD

Exciting new research has emerged focusing on nutrition and its effect on mood. Who would've thought many years ago that what we put in our mouths has a real impact on what goes on in our brains? Lots of recent research has focused on the communication between the gut and the brain, now referred to as the *gut-brain axis*. The gut and brain are connected neurologically by the vagus nerve, which sends signals in both directions. Another way the brain communicates with the gut is through chemical messengers called *neurotransmitters*. Neurotransmitters that are produced in the brain control our feelings and emotions. Serotonin is a neurotransmitter that contributes to our feelings of happiness and also helps control our body clocks. But the brain isn't the only location where serotonin is produced, as 90 percent of our serotonin supply is found in the gut and in blood platelets. Emerging research is showing how the health of the gut and the quality of one's diet can positively or negatively affect mood. In fact, an entire discipline has developed in the world of psychiatry called *nutritional psychiatry*, where medical doctors who have historically treated mental illness with medications and cognitive and behavioral therapies are now adding the power of foods, most importantly plants, to the treatment plan to help those suffering from an array of mental illnesses.

MOOD BOOSTERS

Beans and peas and other legumes
Fermented foods (unsweetened kefir, sauerkraut, kimchi)
Fish

Fresh fruits and vegetables (the more colorful, the better)
Whole grains (avoid packaged and processed foods)
Yogurt without added sugars (contain probiotics and/or live cultures)

PLANTS AND THE ENVIRONMENT

Most of our focus tends to be on how wonderful plants are for our health, but many people don't know the true impact a plant-based diet can have on our environment. Climate change is a real scientific phenomenon that has been at the center of the world stage of alarming global issues. On a daily basis, we experience or are briefed on incidents of extreme weather patterns, sudden outbreaks of diseases, melting of ice caps, disruption of wildlife habitats, and the extinction or near-extinction of various species—all related to the impact of climate change. We are so busy in our lives of consumption that we forget that every second of every day the change in climate has meaningful effects on our living environment and our relationship to the physical world.

Every grade school child now knows common ways to help protect our environment—conserve energy, use less water, recycle, emit fewer toxic gases and chemicals into the environment. It's good that our children are learning these concepts at an early age, as putting measures and practices in place now will be an enormous benefit for them and the world they ultimately inherit. But what many people don't talk about is

how ways in which we grow and eat food can also be important in reducing the emission of environmentally toxic greenhouse gases and their impact on climate.

A report published in the prestigious scientific journal
The Lancet concluded that a global shift from animal to more
plant-based foods is critical to the health of our planet as it re-
lates to reducing greenhouse gases. About 30 percent of global
greenhouse gas emissions comes from food production, and
about half of this is from the livestock sector. Why does this
matter? Methane is one of the most potent atmospheric gases,
warming the atmosphere more than eighty times as much
as the same amount of carbon dioxide does over a twenty-
year period. Cows produce substantial amounts of methane
as part of their normal digestive processes. The amount of
gas emitted is based on the number of animals in a herd, the
type of digestive system they have, and the type and amount
of feed they consume. The more livestock, the more methane they produce during digestion, which means billions of
methane molecules being belched into the air around the
globe every second of every day. If more people around the
world reduce their animal consumption and thus the need for
animal-based food production, this increase in plant-based
eating could reduce death by 10 percent and greenhouse gases
by 70 percent by the year 2050.[6]

It's not just the gas damage to our environment that's a
concern but also the resources we consume in the production
of food. Land use is also a problem. Food production occu-

---

6. Bouvard et al., "Carcinogenicity of Consumption."

pies about 40 percent of the global land. Take a minute and let that number sink in. Almost half of all land on this planet is being used for food production. Yes, we need food to live, but is there not a more efficient way to produce the food so that our nutritional and biological needs are met while we also keep the planet healthy and open so that it can thrive and exist for thousands of years to come? Researchers also look at our fresh water supply, which data has consistently shown is in short supply in many places around the globe. Food production as it stands consumes 70 percent of our fresh water supply, another staggering number that requires a few minutes of reflection to appreciate exactly how substantial a statistic it is.

What do we do next? Understanding this data doesn't mean you have to totally eliminate animal-based products to make a difference; rather, it means you should try at least avoiding the worst climate offenders. The World Resources Institute has listed the offenders by looking at three markers: greenhouse gas emissions, land use, and fresh water consumption. No surprise that beef is by far the worst offender, what many have dubbed an environmental disaster. Following beef on the list is dairy, then poultry, pork, eggs, and fish. In fact, in an effort to reduce climate change through dietary habits, the Intergovernmental Panel on Climate Change (IPCC) has proposed that people reduce their consumption of animal products by 30 percent. Well, after following the Plant Power meal plan in the coming pages, you will be well above that mark, not only improving your health and reducing your risk for many illnesses but helping to keep our planet safe and sustainable for centuries to come.

2

PLANT-BASED:
WHAT
DOES IT MEAN?

Terminology when it comes to nutrition, especially when it deals with diets and styles of eating, can get very confusing. There are many terms and concepts that can mean different things to different people, and even experts don't always agree. However, communication is most productive and effective when terms and concepts are defined so that when they're used, all parties in the discussion can better understand what is being said. (This does not mean they have to agree on the principles, but at least everyone understands the definitions.)

Let's start with my definition of *plant-based diet*.

> A plant-based diet is one that emphasizes plant foods, which occupy a greater percentage of a person's consumption compared to animal-based foods that are consumed in smaller amounts.

There are other definitions that one should be familiar with to be fluent in the language of plant-based conversations.

PLANT-EATING TERMS

VEGAN DIET: a diet that is *entirely* plant-based and excludes anything that comes from an animal, such as meat, fish, dairy, and eggs. (For some, honey is also excluded, as it comes from an insect that they consider as much an animal as cattle.)

VEGETARIAN DIET: a diet that is plant-based and excludes meat but might include dairy and/or eggs (lacto, ovo, lacto-ovo, fruitarian, vegan; a pescatarian also eats fish).

FLEXITARIAN DIET: a mostly vegetarian diet that occasionally includes meat or fish or other animal-based products, but predominantly focuses on plant foods.

PLANT-FORWARD: a style of cooking and eating that puts the emphasis on plant-based foods but is not strictly limited to them. Meat and other animal products might be included, but they are not the central focus of the meal.

PLANT NUTRIENT BASICS

Plants are so powerful because they contain so many important nutrients, most importantly, vitamins, minerals, fiber, and protein. These nutrients help prevent and fight disease, increase our energy levels, help our bodies function better, and help improve our appearance. You can reap the nutritional benefits of plants by eating not only raw and cooked fruits and vegetables but also seeds and nuts. To maximize your plant experience, make sure you consider a wide variety of foods that include fruits, vegetables, legumes, healthy fats, whole grains, plant-based milks, seeds, and nuts. Below, you will find quick reference lists that you can use when shopping for more plant-based items that pack a nutritional punch. These lists are by no means complete but are good examples to help guide your search in the market.

MOST NUTRIENT-DENSE FRUITS

Apples	Lychees
Avocados	Mangoes
Bananas	Olives
Cherries	Oranges
Dragon fruits	Peaches
Durians	Pineapples
Grapefruit	Pomegranates
Grapes	Strawberries
Guavas	Watermelons
Kiwis	

LEGUMES

Beans	Peanuts
Chickpeas	Peas
Lentils	Soybeans

MOST NUTRIENT-DENSE VEGETABLES

Asparagus
Beets
Bell peppers
Broccoli
Brussels sprouts
Carrots
Cauliflower
Collard greens
Garlic
Ginger

Green peas
Kale
Kohlrabi (turnip cabbage or German turnip)
Onions
Red cabbage
Spinach
Sweet potatoes
Swiss chard

HEALTHY COOKING OILS

Canola
Corn
Flax
Grapeseed
Olive

Peanut and other nut oils, such as almond, hazelnut, walnut, etc.
Safflower
Soybean
Sunflower

WHOLE GRAINS

Barley
Brown rice
Buckwheat

Bulgur wheat (cracked wheat)
Corn

Millet	Spelt
Oats	Whole-wheat bread, pasta, or crackers
Popcorn	
Quinoa	100 percent whole-grain breads
Rye	

PLANT-BASED MILKS

(CHOOSE UNSWEETENED OPTIONS)

Almond	Hemp
Banana	Macadamia
Cashew	Oat
Coconut	Rice
Flaxseed	Sesame
Hazelnut	Soy

PLANT-BASED MEAL PROTOTYPE

What should a plant-based meal look like? Does it have to only involve plant-based foods? Can you eat things like pasta? Experts at the Harvard T. H. Chan School of Public Health have written extensively about plant-based diets and their many health benefits. They created a model for what a healthy eating plate should look like as it describes relative portions of fruits, vegetables, healthy oils, proteins, and whole grains.

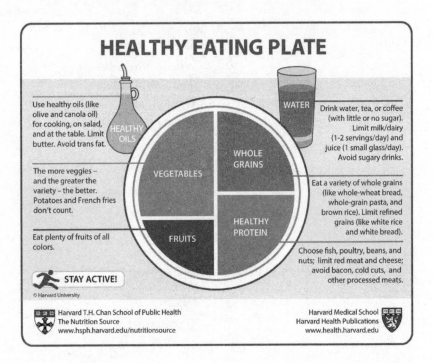

There are some key takeaways that are important to mention when looking at this healthy plate.

1. Notice that half the plate is occupied by fruits and vegetables. This is an easy visual reference as you prepare or order your meals and what comprises them.

2. Whole grains occupy about 25 percent of the plate, and they include whole-wheat bread, brown rice, and whole-grain pasta. This makes it relatively easy to meet your daily suggested intake of whole grains—half your grains should be whole, which means three to five servings.

3. Refined or processed grains, including things like white rice, white bread, cookies, cakes, and other foods made

with white flour, are allowed occasionally but should be kept to a minimum.

4. Healthy protein should comprise 25 percent of your plate. There are great plant-based sources of proteins discussed later in this chapter, but note that animal-based sources such as fish and poultry are included with a suggestion that red meat, cold cuts, bacon, and other processed meats be limited along with cheese (which contains unhealthy saturated fats).

DO YOU NEED TO EAT ORGANIC?

The last ten years has seen a huge boom in the organic food industry, with sales reaching an astounding $50 billion in 2019, according to the 2020 Organic Industry Survey released by the Organic Trade Association. That's almost four times more than organic product sales just fourteen years prior, which only climbed to $13.8 billion. Grocery stores around the country have changed since the early days of organic farming when consumers had to go to small, sometimes out-of-the-way specialty stores to find these specially farmed foods that many believed were healthier and more nutritious. Now you can walk into any major grocery store and find significant shelf space throughout the aisles dedicated to organic products.

But are these organic foods really healthier and more nutritious? The short answer is no. In fact, organic farming was not even started as a mission for healthier food; rather, it began as an effort to help protect the environment. The belief was that traditional farming that used pesticides, fertilizers, hormones, and other chemicals to grow food was damaging the soil and environment. Organic farming was a way to raise crops—both plants and livestock—in the cleanest and purest form without using environmentally toxic chemicals. It is highly regulated by the USDA, with strict standards where the soil is inspected and must be shown to be free of most synthetic pesticides and fertilizers. The crops can't be genetically modified, the livestock aren't given hormones and antibiotics (often used to protect the animals against disease and help guarantee they reach maximal growth), and the feed they're given to eat must have been grown organically. The animals must not be restrictively caged and are free to roam around outside. Practitioners and supporters of organic farming reason that this methodology would not only preserve more of earth's natural resources but would also support the health and continued well-being of animals. While these environmental benefits are absolutely true, that does not mean that the crops themselves are more nutritious. The number of vitamins and other nutrients in an organic banana are the same as those in a conventionally farmed banana. But you will certainly pay more for the organic banana, because the argument is that it's more expensive to organically farm where the manual labor is more costly, profit margins are lower, and farmers lose more crops since they are not using the common chemicals that both help fight crop-killing pests and protect the vulnerable crop until it can be harvested and delivered to your local store.

One argument advocates have made to support the claim that organic crops are healthier is that they have less contamination from pesticides and fertilizers than traditionally farmed crops. However, researchers have studied this extensively and have found that while there might be some chemical residue on these fruits and vegetables, the amount is so small that it poses no real health risks, and the USDA deems these products safe for consumption. For those concerned about the bioaccumulation of the chemical residue over a prolonged exposure (for example, eating lots of fruits and vegetables for many years that might have tiny fractions of chemical residue), there has been no data to raise any concerns about potential negative impact on health.

If you still are worried about the safety of conventionally farmed produce—despite the fact that if there's any real health risk, it's extremely small and can be mitigated by thoroughly washing your produce—and you're willing to shell out a few extra bucks, it might be wise to limit your purchases to those products whose skin you will be eating, since that is where the chemicals, if there are any, will stick. Every year, the Environmental Working Group publishes a list called the Dirty Dozen, which shows the USDA findings of conventionally grown foods most likely to contain pesticide residues. If you want to purchase organic, start with these.

DIRTY DOZEN

Apples	Cherries
Bell and hot peppers	Grapes
Celery	Kale

Nectarines	Spinach
Peaches	Strawberries
Pears	Tomatoes

If you're worried that the meat you're purchasing comes from livestock that was traditionally farmed and might contain hormones and antibiotics, by all means, purchase organic. There still is no compelling data that quantifies how much, if any, of these chemicals remains in the meat you're purchasing in the store or whether their presence will have any negative impact on your health; however, it's everyone's right to be extra cautious. So if you still have concerns and a few extra dollars to spare, splurge on organic meats. While arguments can be made about organic products *potentially* carrying fewer health risks, there are no confirmatory arguments that these foods have higher nutritional quality. An organic lemon has no more nutrients than one that was conventionally farmed, and the last time I checked my local market, the organic version was 30 percent more expensive than one that was conventionally farmed and equal in nutritional value. If you consume enough lemons over the course of the year, that difference adds up to real dollars.

BEGIN YOUR PLANT-BASED JOURNEY

The aim of this book is to help you transition to a more plant-based eating lifestyle. In the following chapters, there is a specific four-week plan to help you make this transition. However, before reading the plan, it helps to mentally prepare yourself with some simple, non-prescriptive things you can do right away to get your mind in the right place and to have a better understanding of the concepts you will be applying on your journey.

EIGHT SIMPLE WAYS TO BECOME MORE PLANT-BASED

LOAD UP ON VEGETABLES: When eating lunch and dinner, make sure half your plate is covered by colorful vegetables. Snacks are also a great way to get in more of those nutrient-packed veggies.

OIL UP WELL: Focus on consuming foods made with good fats. Unsaturated fats are best, so choose things like olive, peanut, soybean, sunflower, canola, flax, corn, safflower, and grapeseed oil.

EXPERIMENT: Try to cook three plant-based entrées every week. Start simple and have an open mind. The more you try and like the recipes, the more you'll be willing to cook them and others.

MEATLESS MONDAYS: Start by agreeing to not eat any meat on Mondays. Every two weeks, add a new day until you are going meatless at least four days of the week.

START WITH SALAD: Incorporate more salads into your regimen and make them the central part of your meal. Experiment with what you put in the salad to increase variety and culinary excitement.

SHOP THE PERIMETER: When you go grocery shopping, make a deal with yourself that more than half the items in your cart will come from the aisles along the perimeter of the store and fewer will come from the aisles at the center.

REPLACE THE PROTEIN: Most of us get the majority of our protein from meat. But plant proteins are equally effective and widely available. Increase the amount of plant proteins and reduce the amount of animal protein.

ACCENT WITH MEAT: Instead of meat being the star of your dish, make it a supporting actor. Use vegetables as the main attraction, but then use a small amount of meat to add texture and taste. Think about a vegetable stir-fry that is predominantly plant-based, but you might add a small amount of beef or chicken.

PLANT PROTEIN POWER

Protein is extremely important to our health and our bodies' functioning. It's one of three macronutrients (carbohydrates and fats are the other two) that the body needs in large supply. Protein is essential in helping to build, repair, and maintain the body's structures. Unlike the other macronutrients, protein is not stored for future use, so we must constantly get it from our diets. Proteins are found throughout the body in muscle, bone, hair, skin, and virtually every other body part or tissue. The thousands of tiny enzymes that power the billions of chemical reactions that occur every second of every day we're alive are comprised of proteins. In fact, at least ten thousand different proteins actually make us who we are.

The National Academy of Medicine recommends that adults get a minimum of 0.8 grams of protein for every kilogram of body weight per day, which is the equivalent of just over

7 grams for every 20 pounds of body weight. For example, a 160-pound adult should consume 56 grams of protein per day. Note that this is just an estimate and there are many factors and medical conditions that influence whether someone should have more or less protein per day, so consulting your doctor is best before deciding what's right for you.

There has been lively debate regarding which is better, animal or plant protein. One important difference between the two involves their amino acid contents. Amino acids are the building blocks of protein such that when the body digests the proteins in food, it breaks them down into these fundamental amino acids. There are nine essential amino acids that make up proteins. Complete proteins are those that contain all nine essential amino acids. Most plant proteins—unlike animal proteins—are incomplete, meaning they are missing at least one of these essential amino acids. There are, however, some plant-based foods that do contain complete protein, and they include amaranth, buckwheat, chia seeds, hemp, quinoa, spirulina, soy, and tempeh.

There is no unanimous opinion about which protein is better, because it really depends on what you're trying to accomplish or the need you're trying to meet. Many believe that animal protein such as whey might give someone trying to build muscle a slight edge, but there is also a belief that rice protein isolate may offer similar benefits to whey. You must also consider that plants contain the very nutritious component of fiber, and animal products don't. Animal products contain the less healthy saturated fat and higher levels of cholesterol than plant-based protein products, so that too should factor into your decision when deciding on which protein best suits your needs. Is animal protein sturdier and certain to help you build and maintain muscle faster? Despite what many have heard or believe, the preponderance of scientific evidence simply does not support this.

SOURCES OF PLANT-BASED PROTEIN

Beans (black, kidney, white, lima)

Brown rice

Chia seeds

Chickpeas

Edamame

Grains

Green peas

Lentils

Nuts (almonds, Brazil, cashews, hazelnuts, peanuts, pine, pistachios, walnuts)

Oats

Quinoa

Seeds (sunflower, pumpkin, hemp)

Spelt

Spirulina

Tempeh

Vegetables (don't contain a lot, but they do contain some)

Wild rice

MEAT SUBSTITUTES AND THEIR CONTROVERSY

One of the hottest debates in the world of nutrition is all the fanfare surrounding meat alternatives or meat substitutes and whether they are healthier than the animal meat products they are meant to replace. One of the original premises behind developing meat substitutes was that reducing meat consumption would mean reducing some of the negative health impacts that come with it. The thinking was straightforward—lower the red meat intake and thus lower the intake of unhealthy substances; increase the plant-based foods and increase the consumption of healthy nutrients.

Based on this and other premises, an entire industry was born, catering to those who wanted to give up red meat and all its associated downsides, yet still wanted to enjoy the taste and texture of meat. It also stood to reason that those whose mission it was to be more environmentally friendly could be satisfied by a more plant-based diet, because it had been shown that land and water use to produce these meat substitutes was significantly less than what was used to produce beef burgers and other meat products.

The biggest concern that researchers and dieticians have raised about the abundance of meat alternatives / substitutes is how they are ultimately manufactured. It's important to understand that it's possible to take something like a plant that is naturally extremely healthy and put it through a manufacturing process that destroys many of its healthy nutrients and replaces them with unhealthy additives that can do more harm than good. For example, the meaty flavor that everyone enjoys in a beef burger can be attributed to a molecule called *heme* that contains iron and is found in the blood. (We humans have the same in our blood—hemoglobin that contains iron and is responsible for carrying oxygen around our bodies.) To re-create this meaty flavor in plant-based burgers, some manufacturers extract heme from the roots of soy plants, then ferment it in genetically engineered yeast. While this trick is effective at producing the appearance and flavor of a beef burger, there's concern that the process produces an even higher intake of heme iron, and this has been associated with increased body iron stores and thus an increased risk of developing type 2 diabetes. Some of these meat alternatives do contain high amounts of plant-based protein, but at what cost? They may also contain a significant number of unhealthy ingredients, including saturated fats and high levels of sodium.

Currently, there is no clear winner in the meatless "meat" trend. It's really a situation of "buyer beware." You need to get beyond the title and healthy-looking packaging and dig into what the ingredients are and where they were sourced. Plant-based "meats" definitely have nutritional and health advantages over red meat, but that's only if they're made from quality ingredients and not crammed with processed "junk." The bottom line is that red meat is what it is, and trying too hard to create something that perfectly mirrors it can not only be extremely challenging but could invite a manufacturing process that introduces ingredients that can be just as unhealthy as what was being avoided in the real meat. Not all substitutes are created equal, so use the shopping guide below to help you make the best decision for your taste buds as well as your arteries.

WHAT TO LOOK FOR IN MEAT SUBSTITUTES

PROTEIN CONTENT: Giving up on animal meat doesn't mean you have to give up protein. There are plenty of substitutes that can keep that protein count high. Look for at least 10 grams of protein per 3-ounce serving.

CALORIE CHECK: Don't assume because it's plant-based that it has fewer calories. Make sure you check the calorie counts and that they fall within the guidelines of what you're looking to achieve.

NUMBERS MATTER: You want a substitute that is not highly processed—consisting of various chemicals and artificial ingredients—as these ingredients can be as harmful as the ones you're trying to avoid in red meat. Typically, the more ingredients a product contains, the more likely the food is processed.

WATCH THE SODIUM: Manufacturers tend to sneak a lot of sodium into these meat alternatives. Aim for a maximum of 250–300 milligrams per serving, as high levels of sodium can put one at risk for high blood pressure. Potassium can help counter the high blood pressure effects of sodium, so check for the amount of potassium, which should be about double that of sodium.

FATS AND SUGARS: Details about these two substances are important to know. Make sure there are low amounts of saturated fats, no trans fats (also listed as *hydrogenated* and *partially hydrogenated oils*), and no added sugars.

OIL CHECK: The types of oil used in these products matter. Look for those products that use unsaturated or polyunsaturated oils, as they are the healthy oils and help lower the LDL (bad) cholesterol. If the product does have some amount of saturated oil, make sure it's less than 2 grams per serving.

3

PLANT
POWER
POINT SYSTEM

The Plant Power Point System allows you to keep track of your animal-based food (ABF) eating in a straightforward and easy-to-track manner. The goal of the transition to mostly plant-based food (PBF) is to go from eating 70:30 animal-based:plant-based to 70:30 plant-based:animal-based. In essence, we are swapping the percentages so that most of what we consume is coming from plants and not animals. For the purposes of our plan, we are not counting honey, even though for many it's considered animal-based.

To make our transition into a plant-based diet easier, we will be using a simple point system that you can track. It all starts with you having 32 total food points over the course of the week. This is how the total points are calculated:

POINT SYSTEM CALCULATION

Meal = 1 point

3 meals × 7 days = 21 meals = 21 points

Snacks (150 calories or less) = 0.5 points*

3 snacks × 7 days = 21 snacks = 10.5 points (round up to 11)

Total Weekly Points = meals + snacks = 21 + 11 = 32 points

*If you consume snacks that are more than 150 calories and contain any animal-based products, then count that snack as 1 full point just as you would a meal.

Let's say you consume 70 percent of your meals and snacks containing some type of animal-based products. That would mean that 70 percent of your 32 points would be categorized as animal-based points. The math is simple. 70 percent of 32 equals 22.4, which we will round down to 22. That means that 22 of your total weekly points are animal-based and 10 points are plant-based. We want to switch those numbers over a gradual four-week span so that 22 of your points will now be plant-based and only 10 points animal-based. This new breakdown will mean that you will still eat animal-based products, but it will be only roughly 30 percent of your diet. This is an attainable goal, and if you achieve this gradually, you will avoid cravings and feelings of deprivation as you transition into more plant foods and fewer animal products.

PLANT POWER

WEEK	WEEKLY ANIMAL-BASED FOOD (ABF) POINTS
One (70% ABF)	22
Two (55% ABF)	18
Three (40% ABF)	13
Four (30% ABF)	10

PLANT POWER POINT SYSTEM ANIMAL-BASED FOOD (ABF) POINTS

FOOD PRODUCT	POINTS
MEAT	
Beef	1
Lamb	1
Pork	1
Veal	1
Organ Meat	1
Wild Meat	1
POULTRY	
Chicken	1
Duck	1
Goose	1
Quail	1
Turkey	1

FISH/SEAFOOD	
All types of fish	1
Anchovy	1
Calamari	1
Caviar	1
Clam	1
Conch	1
Crab	1
Fish Sauce	1
Lobster	1
Mussel	1
Octopus	1
Oyster	1
Scallop	1
Shrimp	1
DAIRY	
Butter	1
Casein	1
Cheese	1
Cottage Cheese	1
Cream	1
Ice Cream	1
Kefir	1
Milk	1
Smoothie (using dairy milk)	1
Whey	1
Yogurt	1
EGGS	
Chicken	1
Fish	1
Quail	1
SNACKS CONTAINING ANIMAL PRODUCTS (150 calories or less)	½
SNACKS CONTAINING ANIMAL PRODUCTS (more than 150 calories)	1

PLANT POWER GUIDELINES

- **Alcohol:** There are no restrictions on alcohol, but it goes without saying that moderation is key. You really should try not to consume more than 1 drink per day on average for women and 1.5 drinks for men. This is based on the typical size difference between the average man and woman. Wines and light beers tend to be healthier choices than mixed drinks, but all alcoholic beverages are at your discretion. If you are trying to lose weight, please note that many alcoholic beverages contain lots of calories that can obstruct your weight loss efforts.

- **Coffee, tea, juices, and other beverages:** These are allowed on the program. It's important to be mindful of what you add to these drinks so they stay healthy and contributive to your efforts to lead a healthier lifestyle. I am not a fan of soda, as it has absolutely no nutritional value whatsoever and is full of chemicals; however, this is a plant-based diet, which means soda is allowed despite my serious recommendations of totally eliminating it or drastically reducing your consumption. Soda and diet soda, regardless of calorie counts, can make the foods they're consumed with taste even better, and thus drinking soda can be a trigger for overeating. You have so much more to gain from healthier drinks, such as teas, fresh juices, and water.

- **Bread:** Bread is considered a plant-based food, as it doesn't contain animal-based products. (Check the ingredients label to make sure.) White bread is allowed, but be mindful that in most cases it tends to be of lower nutritional quality, as the grains used to make the bread have been largely refined (processed) and many of the healthy nutrients have been removed. Some manufacturers try to add back the same nutrients they removed during the processing, so you will see breads that are "fortified" with certain vitamins and minerals; 100 percent whole-grain and 100 percent whole-wheat breads tend to be much healthier and contain less sugar and fewer processed ingredients. Try to make a transition to eating less white bread and more whole-grain breads.

• **Meal switching:** You are allowed to switch meal options within a day or between days as long as they follow the ABF guidelines. If there is a plant-based meal on another day that you want for your current day, it's completely fine to make that substitution. You can do this as much as you like—it's a big part of the flexibility of this program.

• **Weight loss:** While this plan is not specifically meant to be a weight-loss plan, there's no doubt that if you follow it tightly and if you pay attention to portion sizes, there's a very good chance you will lose weight. You can also follow this plan and do intermittent fasting at the same time to increase your chances for weight loss success.

• **Weekly/daily meal plan structure:** The flexibility of the program gives you wide latitude for how you set up your days and weeks. The most important thing is that you stick to the weekly ABF points that are prescribed. You can change which are the ABF meals/snacks within a particular day and even how many ABF meals/snacks there are in a day as long as you don't exceed the weekly total points allowed.

• **Frozen and canned fruits and vegetables:** These are allowed, but please note that in most cases, fresh is better when possible. If you are going to purchase canned or frozen, make sure there's no sugar added and that it's not been loaded with chemicals such as preservatives and other additives involved in processing.

- **Cheese:** When you see that a slice of cheese is allowed, please note that the recommended size is about 3½ inches × 3½ inches. You can choose the type of cheese you want if it's not otherwise specified.

- **Snacks:** For every snack, there are suggestions for you to choose from. You don't have to stick with those listed; you can make substitutions from the snacks chapter or choose snacks that are not in the book as long as they follow the guidelines of what type of snack is called for at that time (ABF versus PBF).

- **Meal/recipe repetition:** You can eat as many of the same foods or prepare the same recipes as often as you like. I highly recommend, however, that you diversify your food choices and try new foods. Diversity keeps things fresh and exciting and prevents food boredom that can lead to you deviating from the plan and eventually falling off.

- **Recipe adjustments:** Feel free to change recipes as necessary. You might have an allergy or food preference or you don't want cheese on your chicken sandwich. No problem—just take it off. As long as you follow the plant-based guidelines when you make your substitutions or eliminations, you are fine.

- **Accelerate the transition:** Maybe you want to eat fewer animal-based foods right from the beginning in week 1. That's not a problem. You can always reduce your ABF points, but you can't increase them beyond the recommended cap for that week.

- **Dairy exceptions:** If you decide to have a dish that is mostly plant-based but has a small amount of dairy (e.g., yogurt spread on toast, 2 tablespoons of cottage cheese, ½ cup milk in your cereal), don't worry about the ABF points. That amount is inconsequential, relatively speaking. If you decide to be a purist, then count them as half a point. But don't beat yourself up about it.

4

PLANT POWER
FIVE-DAY
WARM-UP

Anyone who has lived in a cold climate is acutely aware that during the winter you don't just start your car, shift into drive right away, and take off. You let the engine warm up for a few minutes first; then, once everything is running and the engine seems to have settled, you proceed to shift into gear and drive away. This is the type of approach we will take with the Plant Power meal plan and ultimately your dietary transformation.

The five-day meal plan in this chapter is your warm-up, basically allowing your engine to settle before you take off full throttle on the four-week journey of the meal plan. Use these next five days to get yourself prepared for the transition you're about to undertake. Preparation should be not just physical—what you eat and how you move—but also mental. I have designed this warm-up so that both of these goals can be accomplished, and you will not be jarred on the first week of the full meal plan.

Take a look over the menu items listed for the next five days and decide which options you want for the different meals. Also, make a list of the snacks you'll be eating by using the snacks list in chapter 10. Make sure you choose a combination of plant-based and animal-based snacks as evenly as possible. Once you have made your choices and written them down, you can then create your customized grocery list so that you have all the foods you need to be successful over the next five days. Depending on the meal and snack choices you make, you will also be able to eat out or order in and make those selections accordingly.

Be calm the next five days, open your mind with excitement about this life-changing journey, and most important, *have fun*!

GUIDELINES

- Eat nothing for the first two hours you are awake; nothing to eat within two hours of going to sleep.
- You *must* drink 1 cup (8 ounces) of water before taking the first bite or swallow of your meal; you *must* drink a second cup of water throughout your meal.
- You can have 2 cups of coffee during the day, but they can't contain more than 50 calories total.
- Each day, you must walk/run a total of 10,000 steps (about 5 miles); if you want to do more exercise, all the better, but at least get the 10,000 steps in. All the steps don't have to be completed at one time; you just need to have a total of 10,000 by the end of the day. You can download lots of free fitness apps on your phone that will track your steps.
- You are allowed unlimited plain or fruit-infused water.

- You can swap meals from one day to another, but try to minimize doing that to no more than three times over the course of five days.
- If the menu item listed is something that you don't like or are allergic to or can't access, you are allowed to make swaps, but they must be equal in quality, quantity, and food classification. (You can't swap a cheeseburger for a piece of fish.)
- You can have 1 cup of fresh juice and 2 cups of freshly squeezed lemonade per day.
- Unlimited amount of plain brewed herbal tea allowed per day. (This does not include the ready-to-drink and flavored tea shop choices, because they often contain added fats and sugar.)
- Unlimited spices (salt that's added or in prepared foods must be kept to 1,500 mg or less per day).
- No more than 3 servings of fried foods over the five days.
- For alcoholic beverages, you are allowed 1 mixed drink per day or 2 servings of beer or wine per day. Remember, a serving of wine is 5 fluid ounces.
- Limit your white bread intake, instead choosing more whole-grain or whole-wheat breads.
- *No* white pasta.
- Limit your soda or diet soda intake, or eliminate it entirely.

DAY 1

MEAL 1

Choose one of the following:
- 1 protein shake (350 calories or less, no added sugars)
- 1 fruit smoothie (350 calories or less, no added sugars)
- 2 scrambled eggs with cheese and vegetables

SNACK

- 150 calories or less

MEAL 2

- 1 large green salad with 3 tablespoons vinaigrette dressing (options: 4 olives, 3 ounces shredded cheese, 6 cherry tomatoes, ¼ cup nuts, ½ boiled egg; *no* bacon, *no* croutons, *no* ham)
- 1½ cups soup (options: black bean, white bean, corn, vegetable, tomato, miso, or onion soup)

SNACK

- 150 calories or less

MEAL 3

Choose one of the following:
- 4 servings of vegetables, raw or cooked (a serving size is typically the size of your fist)

- 1 cup cooked whole-grain pasta in a meatless tomato sauce with 1 serving of veggies mixed into the pasta
- 2 cups soup with a small green garden salad (soup options: black bean, white bean, tomato, gazpacho, lentil, chickpea, vegetable, squash, pea, cabbage; *no* creamy or potato soups)

DAY 2

MEAL I

Choose one of the following:

- 1 protein shake (350 calories or less, no added sugars)
- 1 fruit smoothie (350 calories or less, no added sugars)
- One 8-ounce yogurt parfait with low-fat plain Greek yogurt, ¼ cup granola or nuts, and ⅓ cup berries
- 1 fruit plate (3 servings of fruit)
- 1½ cups cold or hot cereal with 1 cup milk and ½ cup berries, or ½ banana, sliced

SNACK

- 150 calories or less

MEAL 2

Choose one of the following:

- 1 large green salad with 3 tablespoons vinaigrette dressing (options: 4 olives, 3 ounces shredded cheese, 6 cherry tomatoes, ¼ cup nuts, ½ boiled egg; *no* bacon, *no* croutons, *no* ham)
- Chicken or turkey sandwich on 100 percent whole-grain or 100 percent whole-wheat bread with tomato, lettuce, and optional cheese and 2 teaspoons of your preferred condiments

SNACK

- 150 calories or less

MEAL 3

Choose one of the following:
- 4 servings of vegetables, raw or cooked
- 1 large green salad with 3 tablespoons vinaigrette dressing (options: 4 olives, 3 ounces shredded cheese, 6 cherry tomatoes, ¼ cup nuts, ½ boiled egg; *no* bacon, *no* croutons, *no* ham)
- 2 small slices pizza with a small green garden salad

DAY 3

MEAL I

Choose one of the following:

- 1 cup oatmeal with fruit of your choice
- 1 fruit smoothie (350 calories or less, no added sugars)
- 1 large fruit plate (for example: ½ sliced apple, ½ sliced grapefruit, 3 slices melon; but any fruit is okay)
- Omelet made with 2 eggs, 3 ounces cheese, and diced veggies
- 2 whole-grain pancakes (5 inches in diameter) with 2 slices turkey or pork bacon and ½ cup berries

SNACK

- 150 calories or less

MEAL 2

Choose one of the following:

- 4 servings of cooked or raw vegetables
- 1½ cups soup (options: black bean, white bean, tomato, gazpacho, lentil, chickpea, vegetable, squash, pea, cabbage; *no* creamy or potato soups)
- 1 large; green salad with 3 tablespoons vinaigrette dressing (options: 4 olives, 3 ounces shredded cheese, 6 cherry tomatoes, ¼ cup nuts, ½ boiled egg; *no* bacon, *no* croutons, *no* ham)

SNACK

- 150 calories or less

MEAL 3

Choose one of the following:
- 4 servings of vegetables, raw or cooked, with 1 cup brown rice
- 2 cups chicken and vegetable stir-fry with ½ cup brown or white rice
- 1 protein shake (350 calories or less, no added sugars)
- 1 large green salad with 3 tablespoons vinaigrette dressing (options: 4 olives, 3 ounces shredded cheese, 6 cherry tomatoes, ¼ cup nuts, ½ boiled egg; *no* bacon, *no* croutons, *no* ham)
- 1½ cups cooked whole-grain pasta in a meatless tomato sauce with 1 serving of veggies mixed into the pasta

DAY 4

MEAL 1

Choose one of the following:

- 1 protein shake (350 calories or less, no added sugars)
- 1 fruit smoothie (350 calories or less, no added sugars)
- 1 large fruit plate (½ sliced apple, ½ sliced grapefruit, 3 slices melon)
- 1½ cups cold cereal with 1 cup low-fat milk and 1 serving of fruit
- One 8-ounce yogurt parfait with low-fat plain Greek yogurt, ¼ cup granola or nuts, and ⅓ cup berries

SNACK

- 150 calories or less

MEAL 2

- 1 large green salad with 3 tablespoons vinaigrette dressing (options: 4 olives, 3 ounces shredded cheese, 6 cherry tomatoes, ¼ cup nuts, ½ boiled egg; *no* bacon, *no* croutons, *no* ham)
- 1½ cups soup (options: black bean, white bean, tomato, gazpacho, lentil, chickpea, vegetable, squash, pea, cabbage; *no* creamy or potato soups)
- 1 meatless burrito (beans, brown rice, guacamole, shredded cheese) in a whole-grain tortilla

SNACK

- 150 calories or less

MEAL 3

Choose one of the following:
- 4 servings of vegetables, raw or cooked, with 1 cup cooked brown rice
- 1 protein shake (350 calories or less, no added sugars)
- 1 cup whole-grain pasta in a meatless tomato sauce with 1 serving of veggies mixed into the pasta
- 6-ounce piece of grilled or baked chicken or fish with 2 servings of vegetables

DAY 5

MEAL I

Choose one of the following:
- 1 protein shake (350 calories or less, no added sugars)
- 1 fruit smoothie (350 calories or less, no added sugars)
- 1 large fruit plate (½ sliced apple, ½ sliced grapefruit, 3 slices melon)
- 1½ cups cold or hot cereal with 1 cup low-fat milk and a piece of fruit

SNACK

- 150 calories or less

MEAL 2

- 1 large green salad with 3 tablespoons vinaigrette (options: 4 olives, 3 ounces shredded cheese, 6 cherry tomatoes, ¼ cup nuts, ½ boiled egg; *no* bacon, *no* croutons, *no* ham)
- 1½ cups soup (options: black bean, white bean, tomato, gazpacho, lentil, chickpea, vegetable, squash, pea, cabbage; *no* creamy or potato soups)
- 1 protein shake (350 calories or less, no added sugars)
- 1 veggie burger on a whole-grain bun with lettuce, tomato, optional cheese, and 2 teaspoons condiments of your choice

SNACK

- 150 calories or less

MEAL 3

Choose one of the following:
- 4 servings of vegetables, raw or cooked
- 1 protein shake (350 calories or less, no added sugars)
- 1 cup whole-grain pasta in a meatless tomato sauce with 1 serving of veggies mixed into the pasta
- 6 ounces grilled or baked chicken or fish with 2 servings of vegetables

5

WEEK ONE

Now that you have completed the five-day warm-up and allowed your car to settle into a good, smooth lane, it's time to push the accelerator down a little. This week is the official beginning of your transition from a mostly animal-based diet to one that is plant-based. I've built a lot of flexibility into the program, so make sure you've read the guidelines in chapter 3 carefully. Follow the meal plan as best you can, but don't get stressed out if you don't hit all the marks. This is a process, and remember that a big part of learning is making mistakes that will teach you valuable lessons. For convenience and clarity, I have marked with (ABF) those meals and snacks that are allowed to have animal-based foods in them. If nothing is marked for a meal or snack, then it's considered to be plant-based only. This pertains to the entire four-week plan. Let's get busy!

DAY I

MEAL I *(ABF)*

Choose one of the following:
- 1½ cups cold or hot cereal with 1 cup low-fat milk
- 2 scrambled eggs with diced veggies and cheese
- 2 whole-wheat pancakes (5 inches in diameter) and 2 slices turkey or pork bacon

SNACK I

Choose one of the following or a plant-based snack from chapter 10:
- 6 cashews
- 12 chocolate-covered almonds or plain almonds
- 1 medium tomato with a pinch of salt
- Black bean salsa over 3 roasted eggplant slices
- 1 cup strawberries

MEAL 2 *(ABF)*

Choose one of the following:
- Chicken or turkey sandwich on 100 percent whole-grain or 100 percent whole-wheat bread with lettuce, tomato, and cheese and 1 tablespoon mustard or mayonnaise
- 5 ounces beef or turkey burger on a whole-grain bun with lettuce, tomato, cheese, and onions and 1 tablespoon ketchup or mayonnaise

THE RISE OF PLANT-BASED EATING

- Plant-based foods are now in 53 percent of U.S. households.
- Thirty-five percent of Americans have consumed plant-based meat in the past year. Ninety percent say they would do so again.
- The number of Americans following plant-based diets is up nearly 9.4 million over the last fifteen years to over 9.7 million in total. However, the number of people who describe themselves as "vegan" or "vegetarian" has changed little and hovers at about 3 percent.
- U.S. retail sales of plant-based foods have increased 11 percent from 2018 to 2019, hitting a plant-based market value of $4.5 billion, outpacing other food sales significantly.
- Internet searches for "plant-based recipes for beginners" increased by 85 percent year over year.

SNACK 2

Choose one of the following or a plant-based snack from chapter 10:

- ⅓ cup wasabi peas
- 6 dried apricots
- 2 stalks celery
- 1 cup grape tomatoes
- 1 kiwi, sliced, with ½ cup oat cereal

MEAL 3 *(ABF)*

- 6-ounce piece of fish (no skin, no frying) with ½ cup brown rice and 1 serving of vegetables
- 6-ounce piece of chicken (no skin, no frying) with ½ cup brown rice and 1 serving of vegetables
- 6-ounce piece of turkey (no skin, no frying) with ½ cup brown rice and 1 serving of vegetables

SNACK 3

Choose one of the following or a plant-based snack from chapter 10:

- 2 frozen fruit bars (no sugar added)
- 3 cups air-popped popcorn
- 10 black olives
- ½ cup quinoa or brown rice
- 5 baby carrots and 3 tablespoons hummus

DAY 2

MEAL 1

Choose one of the following:

- 1 vegan blueberry muffin and 1 serving of fruit
- 1 cup dairy-free chia seed pudding
- Fresh fruit platter with 3 to 4 servings of fruit
- 2 slices 100 percent whole-grain or 100 percent whole-wheat toast spread with 2 tablespoons almond butter

SNACK 1 *(ABF)*

Choose one of the following or an animal-based snack from chapter 10:

- ½ cup low-fat or fat-free plain Greek yogurt with a dash of cinnamon and 1 teaspoon honey
- 1 hard-boiled egg with everything bagel seasoning
- Turkey roll-ups: 4 slices smoked turkey rolled up and dipped in 2 teaspoons honey mustard
- 6 large clams
- 3 crackers lightly spread with organic peanut butter

MEAL 2 *(ABF)*

Choose one of the following:

- 6 ounces chicken breast cooked in a skillet with olive oil, artichokes, garlic, olives, and herbs of your choice
- 1½ cups whole-wheat pasta cooked with marinara meat sauce

- 1½ cups chicken noodle soup or lobster bisque or clam chowder and ½ cup brown or white rice

SNACK 2 *(ABF)*

Choose one of the following or an animal-based snack from chapter 10:
- 6 oysters
- 2 ounces lean roast beef
- Cucumber sandwich: ½ english muffin topped with 2 tablespoons cottage cheese and 3 slices cucumber
- 50 Goldfish crackers
- 1 small chocolate pudding

MEAL 3 *(ABF)*

Choose one of the following:
- 3 beef-and-rice empanadas and a small green garden salad
- 2 small lamb chops with 2 servings of vegetables
- 6-ounce piece of fish or chicken with ¾ cup brown rice and 1 serving of vegetables

SNACK 3

Choose one of the following or a plant-based snack from chapter 10:
- Small baked potato topped with salsa
- ¾ cup roasted cauliflower with a pinch of sea salt
- 1½ cups fresh fruit salad
- ½ large cucumber, cut in sticks or coins, dipped in 2 tablespoons hummus
- 1 cup Cheerios

DAY 3

MEAL I (ABF)

Choose one of the following:

- 1 large salad with 3 ounces fish or chicken sliced on top
- 6-ounce steak with 2 servings of vegetables
- 2 small slices pizza with 2 servings of vegetables

SNACK I

Choose one of the following or a plant-based snack from chapter 10:

- 2 stalks celery and 2 tablespoons organic peanut butter
- 1½ cups fresh fruit salad
- ⅓ cup unsweetened applesauce and ½ cup dry cereal
- 1 medium red bell pepper, sliced, with ¼ cup guacamole
- ½ avocado topped with diced tomatoes and a pinch of pepper

MEAL 2 (ABF)

Choose one of the following:

- 5-ounce beef or turkey burger on a whole-grain bun with lettuce, tomato, cheese, onions, and 2 teaspoons condiments of your choice
- Roast beef sandwich on 100 percent whole-grain or 100 percent whole-wheat bread with cheese, lettuce, tomato, and 2 teaspoons condiments of your choice

- Hummus chicken salad: In a bowl, combine ¾ cup shredded or diced cooked chicken and ⅓ cup hummus. Spread between 2 pieces of 100 percent whole-grain or 100 percent whole-wheat bread.

WATCH THE SODIUM

Consumers need to be careful when they see the words *low sodium, reduced sodium,* and the like. They don't mean anything unless there's context and a clear definition with numbers. Here's a guide to make sure the description matches the true numbers.

LOW SODIUM—contains 140 milligrams or less of sodium per serving

VERY LOW SODIUM—contains 35 milligrams or less of sodium per serving

SALT/SODIUM-FREE—contains less than 5 milligrams of sodium per serving

SNACK 2 (ABF)

Choose one of the following or an animal-based snack from chapter 10:
- 4 turkey slices and 1 medium apple, sliced
- 4 ounces chicken breast wrapped in lettuce and topped with dill mustard
- 7 olives stuffed with blue cheese
- 4 meat-based pot stickers dipped in 2 teaspoons reduced-sodium soy sauce
- Small baked potato topped with salsa

MEAL 3

Choose one of the following:

- 2 small slices pizza with 2 servings of vegetables
- Veggie stir-fry with tofu
- Cauliflower or mushroom steak with sweet potato or roasted sweet potato fries

SNACK 3 *(ABF)*

Choose one of the following or an animal-based snack from chapter 10:

- 1 slice swiss cheese and 8 olives
- ½ cup light natural vanilla ice cream or sorbet
- 1 can water-packed tuna, drained and seasoned to taste
- 10 cooked mussels
- ½ cup canned crab

DAY 4

MEAL 1 *(ABF)*

Choose one of the following:
- 1 serving of frittata (5 inches × 3 inches × 1 inch)
- 2 waffles with 2 slices turkey or pork bacon and 1 tablespoon 100 percent maple syrup
- 1 protein shake made with dairy (300 calories or less, no added sugars)
- Grilled cheese and bacon sandwich on 100 percent whole-grain or 100 percent whole-wheat bread

SNACK 1

Choose one of the following or a plant-based snack from chapter 10:
- 15 frozen banana slices (usually 1 large banana)
- 11 blue-corn tortilla chips
- 2 cups air-popped popcorn
- 2 graham cracker squares and 1 teaspoon organic peanut butter, sprinkled with cinnamon
- ½ cup avocado topped with diced tomatoes and a pinch of pepper

MEAL 2 *(ABF)*

Choose one of the following:
- 1½ cups seafood soup (clam chowder, lobster bisque, fish chowder, bouillabaisse, etc.)

- 2 small slices pizza with a small green garden salad
- Egg salad spread over 1 slice toasted or untoasted 100 percent whole-grain or 100 percent whole-wheat bread (For the egg salad, use 2 hard-boiled eggs, low-fat mayo, dill, mustard, chives, salt, and pepper.)

SNACK 2

Choose one of the following or a plant-based snack from chapter 10:
- 1 medium mango
- 25 frozen red seedless grapes
- 20 medium-size cherries
- 5 tortilla chips and 1/3 cup guacamole
- 1½ cups puffed rice

MEAL 3 (ABF)

Choose one of the following:
- Tomato pesto pasta: Cook 5 halved cherry tomatoes in olive oil in a skillet over medium heat until soft. Mix with 1 cup cooked whole-wheat penne, 2 tablespoons pesto, and diced cooked chicken.
- Shrimp salad: Cook 4 shrimp in a skillet over medium heat, then add ½ cup corn, ½ cup black beans, salt, and pepper. Cook for 3 to 5 minutes, then chill.
- Beef burrito (ground beef or steak, rice, cheese, beans, sour cream) with a small green garden salad

71

SNACK 3

Choose one of the following or a plant-based snack from chapter 10:

- 1 large apple, sliced, sprinkled with cinnamon
- 1½ cups fresh fruit salad
- 6 dried figs
- 20 grapes with 15 peanuts
- Watermelon salad: 1 cup raw spinach with ⅔ cup diced watermelon, sprinkled with 1 tablespoon balsamic vinegar

DAY 5

MEAL 1

Choose one of the following:
- 1 cup Cream of Wheat and ½ cup berries
- 1½ cups cold cereal with 1 cup almond or soy milk and 1 serving of fruit
- Citrus salad: Slice ½ grapefruit and ½ orange into rounds and arrange on a plate. Scoop 2 tablespoons low-fat or fat-free plain yogurt on top and drizzle with 2 teaspoons honey.

SNACK 1

Choose one of the following or a plant-based snack from chapter 10:
- 5 pitted dates stuffed with 5 whole almonds
- ½ cup unsweetened applesauce mixed with 10 pecan halves
- ¼ cup low-fat granola
- 1 cup lettuce drizzled with 2 tablespoons fat-free dressing
- 3 oven-baked potato wedges (baked with cooking spray)

MEAL 2 *(ABF)*

Choose one of the following:
- Tuna avocado salad: Drain 1 can water-packed tuna and combine in a bowl with 2 teaspoons fresh lemon juice,

IAN K. SMITH, M.D.

¼ avocado (mashed), and a pinch of salt and pepper. Scoop the mixture onto a bed of 2 cups leafy greens, cherry tomatoes, ¼ cup red onion slices, and ¼ cup sliced carrots.

- 5-ounce turkey, chicken, or beef burger on a whole-grain bun with lettuce, tomato, onion, and cheese and a small green salad.

- Peanut butter chicken sandwich: Spread 1 tablespoon organic peanut butter on 1 slice 100 percent whole-wheat or 100 percent whole-grain bread, then top with ¼ cup shredded cooked chicken, 1 teaspoon fresh basil or cilantro, and a pinch of salt, and drizzle with extra-virgin olive oil.

THE DOWNSIDE OF ANIMAL PROTEIN

There has been lots of research linking the consumption of red meat to the development of type 2 diabetes. According to NutritionFacts.org, people whose diets were high in animal-based protein (more than 13 percent of calories from animal protein) had seventy-three times the risk of dying from diabetes compared to plant-based eaters. People eating moderate amounts of animal-based proteins (6.5 to 12.5 percent of calories from animal protein) had twenty-three times the risk.

SNACK 2 *(ABF)*

Choose one of the following or an animal-based snack from chapter 10:

- 3 ounces cooked fresh crab
- ½ cup canned crab
- 3 crackers lightly spread with organic peanut butter
- 4 cooked large sea scallops
- ½ cup low-fat cottage cheese with ¼ cup fresh pineapple slices

MEAL 3 *(ABF)*

Choose one of the following:

- 6 ounces citrus-glazed salmon with asparagus and ½ cup brown rice
- 1½ cups zucchini noodles with pesto sauce and 3 ounces diced chicken
- 1 baked pork chop with 2 servings of vegetables

SNACK 3 *(ABF)*

Choose one of the following or an animal-based snack from chapter 10:

- 1 slice swiss cheese and 8 olives
- ½ cup light natural vanilla ice cream or sorbet
- 1 can water-packed tuna, drained and seasoned to taste
- 10 cooked mussels
- ½ cup canned crab

DAY 6

MEAL I *(ABF)*

Choose one of the following:

- 2 waffles with 2 slices turkey or pork bacon and 1 tablespoon 100 percent maple syrup
- 2-egg omelet with diced vegetables and 3 tablespoons shredded cheese or 1 slice cheese
- 1 fruit smoothie (300 calories or less, no added sugars)

SNACK I

Choose one of the following or a plant-based snack from chapter 10:

- 15 frozen banana slices (usually 1 large banana)
- 11 blue-corn tortilla chips
- 2 cups air-popped popcorn
- 2 graham cracker squares and 2 teaspoons nut butter, sprinkled with cinnamon
- ½ cup mini pretzels and 1 teaspoon honey mustard

MEAL 2 *(ABF)*

Choose one of the following:

- Tuna salad sandwich on 100 percent whole-grain or 100 percent whole-wheat bread
- 1½ cups soup (black bean, tortilla, and chicken, or chicken noodle)
- 6-ounce piece of chicken (no skin) or fish with ½ cup rice and 1 serving of vegetables

SNACK 2

Choose one of the following or a plant-based snack from chapter 10:

- ¼ cup almonds
- ½ cup shelled pistachios
- 16 cashews
- 2 medium nectarines
- ½ cup roasted chickpeas

MEAL 3 (ABF)

Choose one of the following:

- 1½ cups cooked whole-grain spaghetti and 3 beef or turkey meatballs the size of a golf ball in marinara sauce
- 2 lamb chops and 2 servings of vegetables
- 6 ounces grilled chicken breast without the skin or baked fish, ½ cup brown rice, and 1 serving of vegetables

SNACK 3

Choose one of the following or a plant-based snack from chapter 10:

- ½ medium avocado sprinkled with a little squeeze of lime juice and sea salt
- 1 medium red bell pepper, sliced, with ¼ cup guacamole
- 21 raw almonds
- 1 cup sugar snap peas with 3 tablespoons hummus
- 10 walnut halves and 1 sliced kiwi

DAY 7

MEAL I *(ABF)*

Choose one of the following:

- 2 pancakes (5 inches in diameter) with 2 slices turkey or pork bacon
- One 8-ounce low-fat yogurt parfait with granola and berries
- 2 scrambled eggs with cheese and ½ cup berries or 1 serving of fruit

SNACK I *(ABF)*

Choose one of the following or an animal-based snack from chapter 10:

- 4 turkey slices and 1 medium apple, sliced
- 4 ounces chicken breast wrapped in lettuce and topped with dill mustard
- 7 olives stuffed with 1 tablespoon blue cheese
- 4 meat-based pot stickers dipped in 2 teaspoons reduced-sodium soy sauce
- Small baked potato topped with salsa

MEAL 2 *(ABF)*

Choose one of the following:

- 5-ounce beef or turkey burger on a whole-grain bun with lettuce, tomato, cheese, and onions and 1 cup french fries

- 1½ cups chili or chicken and vegetable soup or clam chowder and ½ cup brown or white rice
- ½ large burrito (with chicken, steak, or pulled pork and beans, cheese, sour cream) and ½ cup brown rice (Refrigerate and save the other half of the burrito for another meal.)

RED MEAT EXTRAVAGANZA

According to the USDA, the per capita consumption of red meat in 2020 was 111 pounds, which is equivalent to 444 quarter-pound burgers (or 1.2 burgers a day). For context, the World Cancer Research Fund recommends limiting red meat consumption to no more than three 4-ounce portions a week. That means people are eating more than three times the amount of red meat experts recommend as part of a healthy diet. The good news, however, is that this consumption of red meat is less than what it was in 2002 when Americans consumed approximately 125 pounds per capita.

SNACK 2 *(ABF)*

Choose one of the following or an animal-based snack from chapter 10:

- 1 slice swiss cheese and 8 olives
- ½ cup light natural vanilla ice cream or sorbet
- 1 can water-packed tuna, drained and seasoned to taste

- 10 cooked mussels
- ½ cup canned crab

MEAL 3

Choose one of the following:
- 1½ cups cooked whole-wheat pasta with roasted tomatoes and other vegetables if desired
- Vegetarian lasagna (4 inches × 3 inches × 2 inches)
- Black bean burrito with corn, salsa, and guacamole

SNACK 3

Choose one of the following or a plant-based snack from chapter 10:
- Small baked potato topped with salsa
- ¾ cup roasted cauliflower with a pinch of sea salt
- 1½ cups fresh fruit salad
- ½ large cucumber, cut in sticks or coins, dipped in 2 tablespoons hummus
- 1 cup Cheerios

6

WEEK TWO

This week, we are making our first transition step. After starting with 70 percent of our meals being animal-based, we are now going to reduce that to 55 percent. This is not a large decrease, as part of the strategy is that the reduction is real, but it's also not so dramatic that you will feel deprived or crave animal-based foods. The body typically responds much better to changes when they are gradual, giving you the opportunity to adopt this change as a new lifestyle behavior rather than one that is ephemeral and will end up with you reverting to what you were doing before the change. This week, our total ABF points will be 18, which means on average 2.5 ABF points per day. Some days might be a little more and some might be a little less, but the daily average over the course of the week will work out to be 2.5.

DAY 1

MEAL 1 (ABF)

Choose one of the following:

- 2 banana or blueberry pancakes (5-inch diameter) and a serving of breakfast meat (ham or bacon)
- 2 scrambled eggs with 3 tablespoons shredded cheese
- 1½ cups cold or hot cereal with 1 cup low-fat milk and 1 serving of fruit

SNACK 1

Choose one of the following or a plant-based snack from chapter 10:

- ½ cup roasted chickpeas
- Small baked potato topped with salsa
- 3 cups air-popped popcorn
- ½ cup dried apricots
- 1½ cups puffed rice

MEAL 2 (ABF)

Choose one of the following:

- Large salad with 3 ounces chicken or fish sliced on top
- 2 meat tacos with 1 serving of vegetables or a small green garden salad
- 1½ cups chicken noodle soup with ¾ cup brown rice

COW GAS EATS THE ENVIRONMENT

Some studies show that animal agriculture is responsible for 18 percent of global gas emissions, which is more than all forms of transportation combined. Cows and their huge stomachs are the biggest culprits. They produce 150 billion gallons of methane gas per day, which in the short term is far more destructive to the environment than the dreaded villain CO_2 because it has as much as 80 times the warming power as CO_2, even though it only lasts about a decade in the atmosphere, whereas CO_2 can persist for centuries. Think about these numbers as we focus more efforts on reducing CO_2 emissions. That's only part of the answer, as cows will still be belching away and sending all that environmentally toxic methane into the air.

SNACK 2

Choose one of the following or a plant-based snack from chapter 10:

- ¾ cup roasted chickpeas
- ¾ cup roasted black beans
- 3 hummus-and-veggie roll-ups
- 4 dried apricots with 15 dry-roasted almonds
- ½ cup nut-free trail mix with no added sugar

MEAL 3

Choose one of the following:
- Middle Eastern–Spiced Orzo with Charred Eggplant and Peppers (see recipe on page 194)
- 2 cups vegetarian paella
- 4 servings of a variety of roasted vegetables

SNACK 3 (ABF)

Choose one of the following or an animal-based snack from chapter 10:
- 2 tablespoons hummus with 5 baby carrots
- 2 tablespoons hummus with ½ small cucumber, sliced
- 1 whole-grain waffle topped with 2 tablespoons low-fat or fat-free plain yogurt and ½ cup berries
- Hot quesadilla: Spray one side of a corn tortilla with cooking spray, then place in a skillet. Top with ¼ cup Mexican cheese blend, fold in half, and cook for a couple of minutes on each side until the cheese melts and the tortilla is slightly crisp. Serve with 2 tablespoons pico de gallo or salsa if desired.
- 1 small apple, sliced and dipped into ½ cup low-fat cottage cheese and sprinkled with cinnamon

DAY 2

MEAL I

Choose one of the following:

- 1½ cups overnight oats with chia seeds and maple syrup
- Whole-wheat english muffin topped with hummus and avocado slices with 1 serving of fruit
- ½ avocado, mashed and spread on 2 pieces of 100 percent whole-grain or 100 percent whole-wheat toast

SNACK I *(ABF)*

Choose one of the following or an animal-based snack from chapter 10:

- 1 small pear sliced and spread with 1 tablespoon almond butter
- ¼ cup shredded chicken breast served on 5 whole-wheat crackers and topped with 2 tablespoons low-fat shredded cheese and salsa
- Egg and hot sauce sandwich: 1 whole-grain english muffin topped with ½ cup cooked egg whites and drizzled with hot sauce
- Peanut butter chocolate square: 0.4-ounce chocolate square topped with 2 teaspoons creamy natural or organic peanut butter
- 1 sweet apple, such as Golden Delicious or Fuji, with reduced-fat sharp cheddar cheese stick or ¾-ounce slice

MEAL 2 *(ABF)*

Choose one of the following:
- 2 small slices pizza with your choice of topping and a small green garden salad
- 1½ cups chili with ¾ cup brown or white rice
- Turkey or chicken wrap in a whole-wheat tortilla with shredded carrots, lettuce, cheese, tomatoes, and 2 teaspoons of a spread of your choice

SNACK 2

Choose one of the following or a plant-based snack from chapter 10:
- 1½ cups vegan chili topped with avocado slices
- ¾ cup roasted chickpeas
- ¾ cup roasted black beans
- 3 hummus-and-veggie roll-ups
- 1 cup fresh fruit salad

MEAL 3 *(ABF)*

Choose one of the following:
- 6-ounce piece of fish or chicken with ½ cup cooked brown rice and 1 serving of vegetables
- 1 grilled or baked pork chop with 2 servings of vegetables
- 1½ cups whole-grain fettuccine cooked with broccoli, tomatoes, and chicken in a light sauce

SNACK 3

Choose one of the following or a plant-based snack from chapter 10:

- Dehydrated cinnamon apples: Thinly slice 3 medium apples. Sprinkle with cinnamon. Spread evenly on parchment paper in a baking dish. Place in a 170-degree oven for 5 to 6 hours, turning the slices every hour until browned and crispy. (Eat 1 apple's worth of slices as a snack and save the other two for later.)
- 3 tablespoons tomato dip (1 large tomato, ½ teaspoon minced garlic, 2 tablespoons olive oil, and 15 almonds blended in a food processor until smooth) and 4 pita wedges
- Homemade sweet potato chips: Thinly slice 2 sweet potatoes and place in a bowl; mix with 2 tablespoons olive oil and sea salt to taste. Place on an aluminum foil–lined baking sheet and bake in a 375-degree oven for 25 to 30 minutes until desired crispness. (Eat 1 cup of chips and save the rest for later.)
- ½ cup nut-free trail mix with no added sugar
- 2 tablespoons refried bean dip (made without lard) and 5 tortilla chips

DAY 3

MEAL I

Choose one of the following:
- 1½ cups fresh fruit salad with ¼ cup granola
- 1½ cups oatmeal with walnuts, blueberries, and cinnamon
- 2 slices 100 percent whole-grain or 100 percent whole-wheat toast spread with 2 tablespoons almond butter

SNACK I

Choose one of the following or a plant-based snack from chapter 10:
- Organic nut or protein bar (150 calories or less)
- ¾ cup roasted chickpeas
- ¾ cup pico de gallo and 5 tortilla chips
- Black bean salsa over 3 roasted eggplant slices
- 1 cup strawberries

MEAL 2 (ABF)

Choose one of the following:
- 2 ounces ham on 100 percent whole-grain or 100 percent whole-wheat bread with lettuce, tomato, 1 slice cheese, and 2 teaspoons condiments of your choice
- 1½ cups chili and a small green garden salad
- 6-ounce piece of grilled fish with ½ cup rice and 1 serving of vegetables

FIBER AND YOUR HEART

Many studies have looked at the relationship between fiber and heart disease, leading researchers to conclude that a high intake of dietary fiber is linked to a lower risk of heart disease. In a Harvard study of over forty thousand male health professionals, researchers found that a high total dietary fiber intake was linked to a 40 percent lower risk of coronary heart disease; similar findings were found in a study of female nurses.

FIBER: DAILY RECOMMENDATIONS FOR ADULTS

	Age 50 and younger	Age 51 and older
Men	38 grams	30 grams
Women	25 grams	21 grams

SNACK 2 *(ABF)*

Choose one of the following or an animal-based snack from chapter 10:

- ½ cup low-fat or fat-free plain Greek yogurt with a dash of cinnamon and 1 teaspoon honey
- 1 hard-boiled egg with everything bagel seasoning
- Turkey roll-ups: 4 slices smoked turkey rolled up and dipped in 2 teaspoons honey mustard
- 6 large clams

MEAL 3 (ABF)

Choose one of the following:

- Egg and hot sauce sandwich: 1 whole-grain english muffin topped with ½ cup cooked egg whites and drizzled with hot sauce
- 1 whole-grain waffle topped with 2 tablespoons low-fat or fat-free plain yogurt and ½ cup berries
- 1 small apple, sliced and dipped into ½ cup low-fat cottage cheese and sprinkled with cinnamon
- Chocolate graham cracker: Cover 2 graham cracker squares with 2 teaspoons chocolate hazelnut spread and form a sandwich.
- 2 ounces lean roast beef

SNACK 3

Choose one of the following or a plant-based snack from chapter 10:

- ¾ cup roasted chickpeas
- Small baked potato topped with salsa
- 3 cups air-popped popcorn
- ½ cup dried apricots
- 1½ cups puffed rice

DAY 4

MEAL I *(ABF)*

Choose one of the following:
- 2 slices whole-wheat toast with organic peanut butter
- 2 scrambled eggs with spinach, cheese, tomato, and peppers
- 8 ounces low-fat plain Greek yogurt with blueberries and chopped walnuts or pecans

SNACK I

Choose one of the following or a plant-based snack from chapter 10:
- 16 saltines
- ½ cup avocado topped with diced tomatoes and a pinch of pepper
- 21 raw almonds
- ¾ cup roasted cauliflower with a pinch of sea salt
- 10 baby carrots dipped in 2 tablespoons light salad dressing

MEAL 2 *(ABF)*

Choose one of the following:
- Turkey or chicken sandwich on 100 percent whole-grain or 100 percent whole-wheat bread with lettuce, tomato, and cheese and 2 teaspoons condiments of your choice
- Chicken burger on 100 percent whole-wheat bun with

lettuce, tomato, and cheese and a small green garden salad or 1 cup french fries
- 2 small slices pizza with toppings of your choice and a small green garden salad

SNACK 2 (ABF)

Choose one of the following or an animal-based snack from chapter 10:
- 1 fat-free mozzarella cheese stick with ½ medium apple, sliced
- 1 medium red bell pepper, sliced, with 2 tablespoons soft goat cheese
- ½ cup diced cantaloupe topped with ½ cup low-fat cottage cheese
- 3 ounces water-packed tuna, drained and seasoned to taste
- 2 ounces lean roast beef

MEAL 3

Choose one of the following:
- Cauliflower pizza crust topped with pizza sauce, vegan cheese, spinach, and roasted red peppers
- Mushroom, black bean, and avocado enchiladas
- 1½ cups cooked chickpea pasta with marinara sauce and diced vegetables of your choice

SNACK 3

Choose one of the following or a plant-based snack from chapter 10:

- 3 pineapple rings in natural juice, no sugar added
- 2 medium kiwis, sliced
- 3 fresh figs
- 3 to 4 tablespoons dried cherries
- 1 medium grapefruit sprinkled with ½ teaspoon sugar

DAY 5

MEAL I *(ABF)*

Choose one of the following:

- 1 protein shake (300 calories or less, no added sugars)
- 1 waffle with 2 slices turkey or pork bacon and ½ cup berries
- 1 grilled cheese sandwich made with 2 slices cheese on 100 percent whole-grain or 100 percent whole-wheat bread, and 1 serving of fruit

SNACK I

Choose one of the following or a plant-based snack from chapter 10:

- 25 roasted peanuts
- 2 tablespoons pumpkin seeds
- 2 tablespoons shelled sunflower seeds
- ½ cup shelled edamame seasoned with sea salt to taste
- 1 cup radishes, sliced or chopped, drizzled with balsamic vinaigrette

MEAL 2 *(ABF)*

Choose one of the following:

- Turkey or chicken wrap in a whole-wheat tortilla with lettuce, tomato, and cheese and 2 teaspoons condiments of your choice
- 1½ cups Asian beef noodle bowl

- Black bean wrap with avocado, diced tomato, lettuce, and brown rice on a whole-grain tortilla

PLANTS FIGHT CANCER

While cancer treatments have advanced greatly over the years, a tremendous amount of attention has been rightly given to prevention. In some cases, plant-based foods can be a magical elixir, given all the phytonutrients they contain as well as vitamins, minerals, and fiber. Other compounds that have cancer-fighting abilities are alpha-linolenic acid (ALA), lignans, and gamma-tocopherol. The power of whole grains keeps surging along, as some research has shown that eating 6 ounces of whole-grain foods each day may decrease one's colorectal cancer risk by 21 percent.

SNACK 2

Choose one of the following or a plant-based snack from chapter 10:
- ½ cup trail mix with no added sugar
- 3 tablespoons tomato dip (1 large tomato, ½ teaspoon minced garlic, 2 tablespoons olive oil, and 15 almonds blended in a food processor until smooth) and 4 pita wedges
- 4 almond butter–stuffed dates
- 12 chocolate-covered almonds
- 17 pecan halves

MEAL 3 *(ABF)*

Choose one of the following:
- 2 cups turkey chili with ½ cup brown or white rice
- Large salad with 3 ounces steak, chicken, or fish sliced on top
- 1½ cups whole-wheat pasta with vegetables and 3 ounces sliced chicken or fish

SNACK 3

Choose one of the following or a plant-based snack from chapter 10:
- Greek tomatoes: Chop 1 medium tomato and mix with 1 tablespoon feta cheese and a squeeze of lemon juice; add a sprinkle of oregano if desired.
- 1 cup sliced zucchini (roasted if desired), seasoned with salt to taste
- Kale chips: Toss ⅔ cup roughly chopped raw kale with 1 teaspoon olive oil, spread on a baking sheet, and bake at 400 degrees until crisp.
- ¼ cup loosely packed raisins
- 1 pomegranate

DAY 6

MEAL I

Choose one of the following:

- 1½ cups whole-grain cereal with 1 cup oat, soy, or almond milk and 1 serving of berries
- ½ avocado, mashed and spread on 2 pieces of 100 percent whole-grain or 100 percent whole-wheat toast
- 1½ cups overnight oats with fresh fruit
- 3 to 4 servings of fruit

SNACK I

Choose one of the following or a plant-based snack from chapter 10:

- 2 frozen fruit bars (no sugar added)
- 3 cups air-popped popcorn
- 10 black olives
- ½ cup quinoa or brown rice
- 5 baby carrots and 3 tablespoons hummus

MEAL 2 (ABF)

Choose one of the following:

- 1½ cups creamy tomato soup
- 1½ cups chicken noodle soup
- Chicken or turkey club sandwich on 100 percent whole-grain or 100 percent whole-wheat bread with lettuce,

tomato, onion, and cheese and 2 teaspoons condiments of your choice

SNACK 2

Choose one of the following or a plant-based snack from chapter 10:

- ¾ cup roasted chickpeas
- 2 cups watermelon chunks
- 4 dried apricots with 15 dry-roasted almonds
- ½ small apple, sliced, with 2 teaspoons organic peanut butter
- Dehydrated cinnamon apples: Thinly slice 3 medium apples. Sprinkle with cinnamon. Spread evenly on parchment paper in a baking dish. Place in a 170-degree oven for 5 to 6 hours, turning the slices every hour, until browned and crispy. (Eat 1 apple's worth of slices as a snack and save the other two for later.)

MEAL 3

Choose one of the following:

- Whole-grain bowl (1 cup quinoa or brown rice, greens, veggies, drizzled with balsamic vinaigrette)
- Hummus and veggies in whole-wheat pita pocket (1 pita, cut in half)
- 1½ cups vegetable and chickpea stew with ¾ cup roasted potatoes

SNACK 3

Choose one of the following or a plant-based snack from chapter 10:

- White bean salad: ½ cup white beans, squeeze of lemon juice, ¼ cup diced tomatoes, 4 cucumber slices
- ¾ cup roasted cauliflower with a pinch of sea salt
- ½ medium avocado sprinkled with a little squeeze of lime juice and sea salt
- 3 tablespoons tomato dip (1 large tomato, ½ teaspoon minced garlic, 2 tablespoons olive oil, and 15 almonds blended in a food processor until smooth) and 4 pita wedges

DAY 7

MEAL I

Choose one of the following:

- 1 fruit smoothie (300 calories or less, no added sugars)
- 8 ounces soy-based yogurt with granola and strawberries or blueberries (check nutrition label to make sure there isn't a lot of sugar: 5 grams or less)
- 1 cup chia seed pudding with banana slices

SNACK I

Choose one of the following or a plant-based snack from chapter 10:

- 16 saltines
- ½ cup avocado topped with diced tomatoes and a pinch of pepper
- 21 raw almonds
- ¾ cup roasted cauliflower with a pinch of sea salt
- 10 baby carrots dipped in 2 tablespoons light salad dressing

MEAL 2 (ABF)

Choose one of the following:

- 6 ounces salmon with 2 servings of vegetables or a small salad
- Energy bowl: Combine in a bowl ½ cup diced chicken, ½ cup brown rice, ¼ cup cubed cucumber, ¼ cup halved

cherry tomatoes, 2 thin avocado slices, and 2 table-spoons balsamic vinaigrette.
- Greek salad topped with 3 ounces sliced fish or chicken

PLANTS AND YOUR WAISTLINE

People who follow plant-based diets are one step ahead when it comes to shrinking their waistlines. A review of twelve studies that included more than 1,100 people found that those assigned to plant-based diets lost significantly more weight—about 4.5 pounds (2 kg) over an average of 18 weeks—than those assigned to nonvegetarian diets. And for those who do lose weight but struggle to keep it off, eating more plant-based foods might do the trick; the review found that not only did plant-based eaters lose more, but they kept the weight off longer than those who did not follow a plant-based diet.

SNACK 2 *(ABF)*

Choose one of the following or an animal-based snack from chapter 10:
- 1 fat-free mozzarella cheese stick with ½ medium apple, sliced
- 1 medium red bell pepper, sliced, with 2 tablespoons soft goat cheese
- ½ cup diced cantaloupe topped with ½ cup low-fat cottage cheese
- 3 ounces water-packed tuna, drained and seasoned to taste
- 2 ounces lean roast beef

MEAL 3 *(ABF)*

Choose one of the following:
- 6-ounce piece of garlic lemon herb chicken with roasted vegetables and ½ cup potatoes
- 1½ cups whole-wheat pasta with diced chicken or fish
- Grilled or baked pork chop with 2 servings of vegetables

SNACK 3

Choose one of the following or a plant-based snack from chapter 10:
- 1 cup cherries
- 2 small peaches
- ⅓ cup wasabi peas
- 1 large raw carrot
- 1 cup mixed berries

7

WEEK THREE

Congrats on reaching the third week in your transition to a more plant-based style of eating. You should already be experiencing some benefits from eating more plant power foods. Some have reported feeling more energy and less sluggishness, improved skin conditions, and greater mental acuity. This week, we will reduce our animal-based consumption by another 15 percent. This means that your total ABF points this week will be 13. The important part of this week is to focus on how much you are enjoying and learning from eating more plant-based foods. Have you found new dishes that you've eaten and never thought you'd like? Are there certain foods that taste different from what you expected? This week, it's critical to make a mental change and instead of thinking about reducing your animal-based foods, think about increasing your plant-based foods and all the goodness that comes with it. It's not about what you're missing; rather, it's about what you're gaining.

DAY 1

MEAL 1 *(ABF)*

Choose one of the following:

- Greens, eggs, and ham: In a bowl, top ½ cup sautéed kale with ½ cup cooked brown rice, 1 scrambled egg, and 1 slice turkey or pork bacon, chopped.
- Apple toast: Spread 1 tablespoon nut butter of your choice on 1 slice 100 percent whole-grain or 100 percent whole-wheat toast, then top with several thin slices apple and sprinkle with cinnamon.
- Raspberry chia parfait: Mash ½ cup raspberries with 1 tablespoon chia seeds, then add to 8 ounces low-fat or fat-free plain yogurt and top with walnuts or pecans.

SNACK 1

Choose one of the following or a plant-based snack from chapter 10:

- Crispy asparagus: Wash and trim 8 asparagus spears. In a bowl, mix 1½ tablespoons shelled sunflower seeds, ½ teaspoon garlic powder, juice of ½ lemon, ¼ cup whole-wheat bread crumbs, a pinch of ground pepper, and a pinch of paprika. Lay the spears on a baking sheet and evenly cover each spear with the bread crumb mixture. Bake in a 350-degree oven for 20 to 30 minutes until crispy.
- 6 pieces of veggie sushi rolls
- ½ cup small pretzels and 2 tablespoons hummus

- ½ cup cooked organic instant oatmeal with berries
- 20 organic seaweed snacks

MEAL 2 *(ABF)*

Choose one of the following:

- Chicken lettuce wraps: In a bowl, combine 3 ounces cooked chicken, ½ cup chopped pecans, ⅓ cup chopped red bell pepper, ⅓ cup shredded carrot, and 2 tablespoons hummus. Spread the mixture on 2 whole romaine lettuce leaves.
- Cashew cucumber salad: In a bowl, mix 1 small cucumber, peeled and diced, ½ cup diced tomatoes, ½ cup cashews, juice of ½ lime, 1 tablespoon olive oil, and a pinch each of salt and pepper.
- Meatball soup: Cook 3 turkey or beef meatballs the size of a golf ball and add to 1½ cups hot vegetable soup.

SNACK 2

Choose one of the following or a plant-based snack from chapter 10:

- Organic nut or protein bar (150 calories or less)
- 1 baked tofu bar
- 2 scoops of sorbet
- ½ cup roasted lupini beans
- ¼ cup cashews with ¼ cup dried cranberries

MEAL 3

Choose one of the following:

- Oven-Roasted Mushroom, Artichoke, and Dandelion Greens Salad (see recipe on page 198)
- 4 servings roasted vegetables with 1 cup cooked brown rice
- 2 cups vegetable stir-fry using veggies of your choice

SNACK 3

Choose one of the following or a plant-based snack from chapter 10:

- 3 cups air-popped popcorn
- 1 cup baked apple chips
- Plant-based crackers (150 calories or less)
- 1 fruit bar
- 1 stalk celery cut into sections and 2 tablespoons nut butter

DAY 2

MEAL 1 (ABF)

Choose one of the following:

- 2 slices of french toast made with 100 percent whole-grain or 100 percent whole-wheat bread and ½ cup berries
- ¾ cup bran flakes with sliced banana, blueberries, and reduced-fat milk
- Bacon grilled cheese sandwich: Butter one side of 2 pieces of 100 percent whole-grain or 100 percent whole-wheat bread, then set aside. Cook 3 slices turkey or pork bacon. Place 1 piece of bread, buttered side down, in a skillet over medium heat. Place a piece of cheese on top of the bread, then cut the bacon strips in half and place on top of the cheese. Place a second piece of cheese on top of the bacon, then put the second piece of bread on top to complete the sandwich. Make sure the buttered side is facing up. Cook until golden brown and the cheese is melting, then flip and cook on the second side.

SNACK 1

Choose one of the following or a plant-based snack from chapter 10:

- 5 pitted dates stuffed with 5 whole almonds
- ½ cup unsweetened applesauce mixed with 10 pecan halves
- ¼ cup low-fat granola

- 40 shelled pistachios
- ¾ cup melon cubes

MEAL 2

Choose one of the following:
- 1½ cups black bean soup and a small green garden salad
- 1½ cups pea soup and a small green garden salad
- 1½ cups lentil soup and a small green garden salad

PLANT-BASED MILKS SAVE THE PLANET

The enormous use of water in raising, breeding, and processing cattle is well documented and has become a rallying cry for many environmentalists. Some of their answers to protecting the environment can be found in plant-based milks. Some estimates report that substituting almond milk for cow's milk conserves as much as 40 gallons of water per 1 cup of milk substituted. When it comes to plant-based milks, soy and oat milk get the gold star, with rice and almond milk still doing better than dairy, but they are not as water-conserving as soy and oat. Beyond the water conservation, these milks also can help reduce greenhouse gas emissions. Cow's milk can be responsible for more than triple the CO_2 emissions compared to almond and soy milk.

TYPE OF MILK	WATER USE (GALLONS)
Cow	166
Almond	98
Rice	71
Oat	13
Soy	7

SNACK 2 *(ABF)*

Choose one of the following or an animal-based snack from chapter 10:

- Open-faced turkey swiss melt: On half of a whole-wheat english muffin, place ¾ ounce low-sodium deli turkey and 1 thin slice swiss cheese. Melt and serve.
- Peanut butter chocolate square: 0.4-ounce chocolate square topped with 2 teaspoons creamy natural or organic peanut butter
- 1 sweet apple, such as Golden Delicious or Fuji, with reduced-fat sharp cheddar cheese stick or ¾-ounce slice
- 7 olives stuffed with 1 tablespoon blue cheese
- 4 meat-based pot stickers dipped in 2 teaspoons reduced-sodium soy sauce

MEAL 3

Choose one of the following:

- Fusilli with Green Beans, Tomatoes, and Toasted Garlic (see recipe on page 188)
- Spicy Thai Vegetable Stir-Fry (see recipe on page 214)
- Roasted Grape, Endive, and Bulgur Salad with Feta (see recipe on page 206)
- Large salad (all or any of the following: ½ cup beans, 3 cups lettuce or other greens, 5 olives, 3 tablespoons shredded cheese, 5 cherry tomatoes, 2 tablespoons nuts, sliced cucumbers) with 2 tablespoons low-fat or fat-free vinaigrette-type dressing

SNACK 3 *(ABF)*

Choose one of the following or an animal-based snack from
chapter 10:

- 5 whole-grain crackers with mini Gouda cheese round
- 10 baby carrots with ½ cup cottage cheese that's been
  mixed with ½ tablespoon pesto sauce
- Yogurt-dipped strawberries: Dip 1 cup of whole strawberries in ½ cup low-fat vanilla Greek yogurt, place on a
  baking sheet, and freeze.
- 1 cup 2 percent ultra-filtered chocolate milk
- Honey-ricotta rice cake: Spread 3 tablespoons ricotta
  cheese over 1 brown rice cake, then drizzle with 2 teaspoons honey.

DAY 3

MEAL I (ABF)

Choose one of the following:
- Avocado toast with sunflower seeds: Spread ½ avocado on 1 slice 100 percent whole-grain or 100 percent whole-wheat toast, then top with 2 small slices tomato and 1 tablespoon shelled sunflower seeds.
- Raspberry chia parfait: Mash ½ cup raspberries with 1 tablespoon chia seeds, then add to 8 ounces low-fat or fat-free plain yogurt and top with walnuts or pecans.
- 2 scrambled eggs with optional cheese and 2 small turkey or pork sausage links or 2 strips turkey or pork bacon. Eat with 1 serving of fruit of your choice.

SNACK I

Choose one of the following or a plant-based snack from chapter 10:
- 3 pineapple rings in natural juice, no sugar added
- 10 baby carrots dipped in 2 tablespoons light salad
- dressing
- White bean salad: ⅓ cup white beans, squeeze of lemon juice, ¾ cup diced tomatoes, 4 cucumber slices
- 1 nectarine
- 3 to 4 tablespoons dried cherries

MEAL 2

Choose one of the following:

- Artichoke and Chickpea Caesar Salad (see recipe on page 154)
- Black bean wrap with avocado, diced tomato, lettuce, and brown rice on a whole-grain tortilla
- Large salad (all or any of the following: lettuce, 5 olives, 3 tablespoons shredded cheese, 5 cherry tomatoes, 2 tablespoons nuts, sliced cucumbers) with 2 tablespoons low-fat or fat-free vinaigrette-type dressing

SNACK 2

Choose one of the following or a plant-based snack from chapter 10:

- 8 to 10 slices cucumber and 2 tablespoons hummus
- Watermelon and honeydew melon balls (8 total)
- 1 slice 100 percent whole-wheat bread or 1 whole-grain pita pocket, cut into quarters, with 2 tablespoons hummus
- 2 cups air-popped popcorn drizzled with a rosemary-lemon combo made from combining and heating 2 teaspoons olive oil, 2 teaspoons minced rosemary, ¼ teaspoon grated lemon zest, and a pinch of sea salt
- Homemade trail mix: Combine 7 roasted almonds, 2 tablespoons dried cranberries, 5 mini pretzel twists, and 1 tablespoon shelled sunflower seeds.

MEAL 3 *(ABF)*

Choose one of the following:

- 6-ounce piece of grilled or baked fish with 2 servings of vegetables
- 6-ounce piece of grilled or baked chicken breast (no skin) with 2 servings of vegetables
- 1 piece of layered meat lasagna (4 inches × 3 inches × 2 inches) with a small garden salad or 2 servings of vegetables

SNACK 3

Choose one of the following or a plant-based snack from chapter 10:

- 16 saltines
- ½ cup avocado topped with diced tomatoes and a pinch of pepper
- 21 raw almonds
- 20 frozen grapes
- Sweet walnut oatmeal (½ cup cooked steel-cut oats topped with 1 tablespoon chopped walnuts and drizzled with 1 teaspoon organic honey or 100 percent maple syrup)

DAY 4

MEAL I

Choose one of the following:

- Green smoothie: Combine ½ cup peeled chopped apple with 4 chopped kale leaves, ½ cup chopped mango, ¾ cup water, and ½ cup low-fat or fat-free plain yogurt in a blender and purée on low speed.
- 1 vegan blueberry or corn muffin with 1 serving of fruit
- 1½ cups hot or cold cereal with 1 cup nondairy milk of your choice and a serving of fruit

SNACK I

Choose one of the following or a plant-based snack from chapter 10:

- ½ cup sweet potato chips
- 6 dried apricots with 1 tablespoon dried cherries
- Small kale salad: 1 cup kale leaves topped with ¾ cup roasted chickpeas and drizzled with tahini dressing
- 15 frozen banana slices (usually 1 large banana)
- 11 blue-corn tortilla chips

MEAL 2 (ABF)

Choose one of the following:

- Chicken bowl: Toss 2 cups greens of your choice with 3 ounces diced grilled chicken, ¼ cup diced apple, ¼ cup shredded carrots, 2 tablespoons hummus, and 1 tablespoon lemon juice.

- Cucumber tuna salad: Drain 1 can of tuna, then place in a bowl and mix in ½ cup peeled and diced cucumbers, ½ tablespoon fresh lemon juice, 1 tablespoon mayonnaise, and a pinch of salt. Serve on a bed of greens or inside a whole-wheat tortilla.
- Power salmon bowl: In a bowl, place 2 cups chopped greens of your choice, 3 ounces chopped cooked salmon, ½ cup diced cucumbers, ¼ cup shredded carrots, ½ cup diced tomatoes, and ½ cup cooked brown rice. Drizzle with balsamic vinaigrette.

MIND YOUR VITAMINS

Vital nutrients such as vitamin D, omega-3 fatty acids, and iron are more difficult to find in plant-based sources compared to their animal counterparts. Vitamin B_{12}, which is vital for energy production, our blood circulation systems, and our nervous systems, is not available at all in plants but naturally available only in animals. Plant-based eaters can still get their vitamin B_{12} by consuming B_{12}-fortified products, such as plant-based milk, various dairy products, and meat alternatives.

SNACK 2 (ABF)

Choose one of the following or an animal-based snack from chapter 10:
- 6 cucumber, cherry tomato, and mozzarella ball skewers
- 6 pieces of spicy tuna sushi rolls
- 2 ounces beef or turkey jerky

- 4 chocolate chip cookies, each a little larger than the size of a poker chip
- Turkey-wrapped avocado: ¼ avocado sliced and wrapped in 3 ounces low-sodium deli turkey meat

MEAL 3

Choose one of the following:
- Arugula Salad with Roasted New Potatoes and Pickled Pepper Dressing (see recipe on page 157)
- 1½ cups polenta topped with roasted eggplant, mushrooms, and red peppers
- Kale and squash salad topped with dressing of your choice

SNACK 3 *(ABF)*

Choose one of the following or an animal-based snack from chapter 10:
- 1 medium red bell pepper, sliced, with 2 tablespoons soft goat cheese
- Grilled portobello mushroom stuffed with roasted vegetables and 1 teaspoon shredded cheese
- 1 ounce cheddar cheese with 5 radishes
- Cucumber sandwich: ½ english muffin topped with 2 tablespoons cottage cheese and 3 slices cucumber
- 1 hard-boiled egg and ½ cup sugar snap peas
- 3 ounces cooked fresh crab

DAY 5

MEAL I

Choose one of the following:

- 1 cup Cream of Wheat and ½ cup berries
- 1½ cups cold cereal with 1 cup almond or soy milk and 1 serving of fruit
- Citrus salad: Slice ½ grapefruit and ½ orange into rounds and arrange on a plate. Scoop 2 tablespoons low-fat or fat-free plain yogurt on top and drizzle with 2 teaspoons organic honey.

SNACK I

Choose one of the following or a plant-based snack from chapter 10:

- 20 grapes with 15 peanuts
- Watermelon salad: 1 cup raw spinach with ⅔ cup diced watermelon, sprinkled with 1 tablespoon balsamic vinegar
- ¾ cup roasted chickpeas
- ¾ cup roasted black beans
- ½ grapefruit sprinkled with ½ teaspoon sugar

MEAL 2 (ABF)

Choose one of the following:

- 1½ cups beef and vegetable stew with ½ cup white or brown rice

- Ham roll-ups: Spread blue cheese salad dressing on one side of 2 slices of deli ham. Top with several thin slices cucumber. Roll up each piece of ham and serve on a bed of greens.
- 2 small slices pizza with toppings of your choice and a small green garden salad

SNACK 2

Choose one of the following or a plant-based snack from chapter 10:
- 4 dried apricots with 15 dry-roasted almonds
- 1 cup fresh fruit salad
- ¾ cup pico de gallo and 5 tortilla chips
- 4 almond butter–stuffed dates
- 3 cups air-popped popcorn

MEAL 3 *(ABF)*

Choose one of the following:
- 1½ cups cooked whole-grain spaghetti and 3 turkey or beef meatballs the size of a golf ball in marinara sauce
- Chicken stir-fry: Cook 6-ounce chicken breast, dice, then set aside. Add ¼ cup diced red bell peppers, ¼ cup diced tomatoes, 1 tablespoon diced onion, 1 teaspoon minced garlic, and a pinch each of salt and pepper to the skillet. Cook the vegetables for about 5 minutes, stirring frequently. Return the chicken to the skillet and cook for another couple of minutes until heated through.

- 6-ounce piece of chicken or fish with 2 servings of vege-tables

SNACK 3

Choose one of the following or a plant-based snack from chapter 10:

- ⅓ cup loosely packed raisins
- 1 cup strawberries
- 2 Popsicles
- 50 Goldfish crackers
- 2 tablespoons hummus spread on 4 crackers

DAY 6

MEAL I

Choose one of the following:

- Apple toast: Spread 1 tablespoon nut butter of your choice on 1 slice 100 percent whole-grain or 100 percent whole-wheat toast, then top with several thin slices of apple and sprinkle with cinnamon
- ¾ cup bran flakes with sliced banana, blueberries, and nondairy milk
- 1 fruit smoothie (300 calories or less, no added sugars)

SNACK I *(ABF)*

Choose one of the following or an animal-based snack from chapter 10:

- ¼ cup cantaloupe topped with ½ cup low-fat cottage cheese
- 1 cup fresh red raspberries topped with ½ cup low-fat yogurt
- 1 medium red bell pepper, sliced, with 2 tablespoons soft goat cheese
- 5 cucumber slices topped with ⅓ cup cottage cheese, salt, and pepper
- 1 can water-packed tuna, drained and seasoned to taste

MEAL 2

Choose one of the following:

- Fennel, Celery Root, and Apple Salad with Pita Croutons (see recipe on page 184)
- Quinoa bowl with roasted carrots and sweet potatoes
- 1½ cups vegetable soup and ¾ cup brown rice

FEED THE BUGS

Your gastrointestinal tract is lined with bacteria that live there and keep you healthy. This is called our *microbiome* and can weigh as much as five pounds, which means billions and billions of bacteria. These bacteria do many things, including digest food, regulate our immune systems, produce vitamins, and fight bad bacteria that invade us. These bacteria, just like our bodies' cells, need to be fed. Soluble fiber is their preferred fuel source, which is another reason to make sure you're eating enough daily fiber.

SNACK 2 *(ABF)*

Choose one of the following or an animal-based snack from chapter 10:

- 2 tablespoons hummus with 5 baby carrots
- 2 tablespoons hummus with ½ small cucumber, sliced
- 1 slice swiss cheese and 8 olives

- ½ cup light natural vanilla ice cream or sorbet
- 1 can water-packed tuna, drained and seasoned to taste

MEAL 3 *(ABF)*

Choose one of the following:
- Tuna burgers: Drain a can of water-packed tuna and combine in a bowl with 1 egg, beaten, ½ teaspoon garlic powder, ½ teaspoon turmeric, ½ teaspoon onion powder, and a pinch each of salt and pepper. Make 2 patties and cook in a skillet in olive oil until crispy. Eat with 2 servings of vegetables or a small green garden salad.
- 1½ cups whole-grain pasta with meat sauce and a serving of vegetables
- 6-ounce piece of grilled or baked fish or chicken with 2 servings of vegetables

SNACK 3 *(ABF)*

Choose one of the following or an animal-based snack from chapter 10:
- Open-faced turkey swiss melt: On half of a whole-wheat english muffin, place ¾ ounce low-sodium deli turkey and 1 thin slice swiss cheese. Melt and serve.
- Tomato-mozzarella salad: Cube 1 ounce fresh mozzarella and combine in a small bowl with 11 halved cherry tomatoes and 2 teaspoons chopped fresh basil, then drizzle with 1 tablespoon balsamic vinaigrette.
- 4 turkey slices and 1 medium apple, sliced

- 2 hard-boiled eggs with a pinch each of salt and pepper
- Chocolate-dipped pretzels: Melt 1 tablespoon semisweet chocolate morsels in a microwave. Dip 3 honey pretzel sticks in the chocolate. Put the pretzels in the freezer until the chocolate sets.

DAY 7

MEAL I *(ABF)*

Choose one of the following:

- 2 pancakes (5 inches in diameter) with 2 slices turkey or pork bacon
- 2 scrambled eggs with optional cheese and 2 small sausage links or 2 slices turkey or pork bacon. Eat with 1 serving of fruit of your choice.
- 2 slices french toast made with 100 percent whole-grain or 100 percent whole-wheat bread and ½ cup berries

SNACK I

Choose one of the following or a plant-based snack from chapter 10:

- ⅓ cup unsweetened applesauce and ½ cup dry cereal
- 1 medium red bell pepper, sliced, with ¼ cup guacamole
- ½ cup avocado topped with diced tomatoes and a pinch of pepper
- ¾ cup roasted black beans
- Small garden salad (greens, tomatoes, olives, shredded carrots)

MEAL 2

Choose one of the following:

- Cucumber, Watermelon, and Avocado Salad with Chili-Mint Vinaigrette (see recipe on page 181)

- 1½ cups soup (tomato, pea, mushroom, or lentil) and ¾ cup cooked brown rice
- Large salad (all or any of the following: ½ cup beans, 3 cups lettuce or other greens, 5 olives, 3 tablespoons shredded cheese, 5 cherry tomatoes, 2 tablespoons nuts, sliced cucumbers) with 2 tablespoons low-fat or fat-free vinaigrette-type dressing

SNACK 2 *(ABF)*

Choose one of the following or an animal-based snack from chapter 10:

- 1 slice swiss cheese and 8 olives
- ½ cup light natural vanilla ice cream or sorbet
- 1 can water-packed tuna, drained and seasoned to taste
- 10 cooked mussels
- ½ cup canned crab

MEAL 3 *(ABF)*

Choose one of the following:

- Chicken stir-fry: Cook 6-ounce chicken breast, dice, then set aside. Add ¼ cup diced red bell peppers, ¼ cup diced tomatoes, 1 tablespoon diced onion, 1 teaspoon minced garlic, and a pinch each of salt and pepper to the skillet. Cook the vegetables for about 5 minutes, stirring frequently. Return the chicken to the skillet and cook for another couple of minutes until heated through.
- Large salad (all or any of the following: ½ cup beans, 3 cups lettuce or other greens, 5 olives, 3 tablespoons shredded cheese, 5 cherry tomatoes, 2 tablespoons nuts,

sliced cucumbers) with 2 tablespoons low-fat or fat-free vinaigrette-type dressing, topped with 3 ounces fish or chicken
- 3 giant crab legs with butter sauce dip and 2 servings of vegetables

SNACK 3

Choose one of the following or a plant-based snack from chapter 10:
- ⅓ cup unsweetened applesauce and ½ cup dry cereal
- 10 walnut halves and 1 sliced kiwi
- Baby burrito: Spread 2 tablespoons bean dip on a 6-inch corn tortilla and top with 2 tablespoons salsa.
- 1 cup grapes with 10 almonds
- 5 pieces of brown rice vegetable sushi rolls

8

WEEK FOUR

You have finally arrived! You are now predominantly plant-based. Depending on how dependent you previously were on animal-based foods, this will be quite an achievement. I designed the Plant Power plan to make your transition to this point as smooth as possible. Many people will reach this week and decide to go fully plant-based, which means becoming a vegan or vegetarian. Others will decide that they occasionally want to consume animal-based foods as a smaller portion of their diet, and this is what this last week represents. It's something you can easily do for the rest of your life if you choose to.

This week completes the full conversion to a new 70:30 plant-based:animal-based ratio. Your total ABF points for the week will now be reduced to 10. There are many ways to reach these 10 points over the course of seven days. The week that I have listed here, similar to the others, is just a suggestion. The beauty of using a point system is that *you* can ultimately decide how you configure your week as long as you don't surpass the total of 10 ABF points. Do whatever works for you, but most of all, be excited that you are now fueling your body in a way that will maximize disease prevention, increase longevity, and help you achieve peak performance.

DAY 1

MEAL 1 *(ABF)*

Choose one of the following:

- Open-faced egg sandwich: On a whole-grain english muffin or slice of bread, place ⅓ cup cooked sautéed spinach over 1 cooked egg, sprinkle 1 tablespoon shredded cheese, and season with salt and pepper to taste. Eat with 1 serving of fruit of your choice.
- 2 whole-wheat pancakes (5 inches in diameter), 2 slices turkey or pork bacon, and 1 serving of fruit
- 1 protein shake (300 calories or less, no added sugars)

SNACK 1

Choose one of the following or a plant-based snack from chapter 10:

- Small baked potato topped with salsa
- ¾ cup roasted cauliflower with a pinch of sea salt
- 1½ cups fresh fruit salad
- ⅓ cup unsweetened applesauce and ½ cup dry cereal
- 1 medium red bell pepper, sliced, with ¼ cup guacamole

MEAL 2

Choose one of the following:

- Crispy Zucchini Fingers with Green Goddess Dip (see recipe on page 177)

- 1½ cups black bean soup, white bean soup, or vegan chili with ¾ cup brown rice
- Large salad (all or any of the following: ½ cup beans, 3 cups lettuce or other greens, 5 olives, 3 tablespoons shredded cheese, 5 cherry tomatoes, 2 tablespoons nuts, sliced cucumbers) with 2 tablespoons low-fat or fat-free vinaigrette-type dressing

DON'T FORGET YOUR CALCIUM

Calcium is one of the most important minerals for our bodies, essential for strong bones and teeth as well as for our muscles to be able to move and our nerves to send electrical signals. The amount of calcium one needs depends on gender and age. Dairy foods are loaded with calcium, but if you're not eating much dairy, then you will need to find calcium from other sources, such as leafy green vegetables, nuts, red kidney beans, soy, sesame seeds, dried fruit, and fortified plant-based dairy.

MEN	
19–50 years	1,000 mg/day
51–70 years	1,000 mg/day
71 and older	1,200 mg/day

WOMEN	
19–50 years	1,000 mg/day
51 and older	1,200 mg/day

SNACK 2 *(ABF)*

Choose one of the following or an animal-based snack from chapter 10:

- ½ cup pudding of your choice
- 3 celery sticks stuffed with cottage cheese (each stick should be 5 inches long)
- 1 portobello mushroom stuffed with roasted veggies and 1 teaspoon shredded low-fat cheese
- 8 small shrimp and 2 tablespoons cocktail sauce
- 1 cup chicken noodle soup

MEAL 3

Choose one of the following:

- Barley with Crispy Brussels Sprouts, White Beans, and Browned Butter Vinaigrette (see recipe on page 159)
- 2 spicy peanut lettuce wraps filled with baked tofu, carrots, cucumbers, peppers, and roasted cauliflower
- 1 black bean enchilada and a small garden salad

SNACK 3

Choose one of the following or a plant-based snack from chapter 10:

- ½ cup dried apricots
- 1½ cups puffed rice
- Watermelon salad: 1 cup raw spinach with ⅔ cup diced watermelon, sprinkled with 1 tablespoon balsamic vinegar
- 25 frozen red seedless grapes

DAY 2

MEAL I

Choose one of the following:

- 1½ cups overnight oats with fresh fruit
- Apple toast: Spread 2 slices 100 percent whole-grain or 100 percent whole-wheat bread with nut butter and top with thin slices of Granny Smith apple.
- Strawberry toast: Spread 1 slice 100 percent whole-grain or 100 percent whole-wheat bread with 2 tablespoons plain Greek yogurt, 2 thinly sliced strawberries, and ½ teaspoon balsamic reduction.

SNACK I

Choose one of the following or a plant-based snack from chapter 10:

- ½ cup avocado topped with diced tomatoes and a pinch of pepper
- ¾ cup roasted black beans
- Small garden salad (greens, tomatoes, olives, shredded carrots)
- ⅓ cup unsweetened applesauce and ½ cup dry cereal
- 4 almond butter–stuffed dates

MEAL 2 (ABF)

Choose one of the following:

- Beef burrito bowl: Combine 2 cups brown rice, 1 cup beans of your choice, 3 ounces beef, ½ small avocado,

131

sliced, ⅓ cup shredded lettuce, and 2 tablespoons diced onions.

- 8 spicy shrimp with ½ cup brown rice and 1 serving of vegetables
- Crème cucumber salad: In a medium bowl, mix 1 small cucumber, peeled and diced, with ⅓ cup diced chicken, 2 tablespoons mayo, and a pinch each of salt and pepper.

SNACK 2

Choose one of the following or a plant-based snack from chapter 10:

- 1 cup sugar snap peas with 3 tablespoons hummus
- 10 walnut halves and 1 sliced kiwi
- 5 pitted dates stuffed with 5 whole almonds
- ¾ cup steamed edamame
- ½ cup pretzels and 1 teaspoon honey mustard

MEAL 3

Choose one of the following:

- Pearl Couscous with Summer Squash, Cherry Tomatoes, and Pistachio Vinaigrette (see recipe on page 202)
- Meat-stuffed peppers: Hollow out two halves of a red bell pepper, load each half with cooked ground beef, then top with cheese and put into the oven on low heat until the cheese melts.
- Large salad (all or any of the following: ½ cup beans, 3 cups lettuce or other greens, 5 olives, 3 tablespoons shredded cheese, 5 cherry tomatoes, 2 tablespoons nuts,

sliced cucumbers) with 2 tablespoons low-fat or fat-free vinaigrette-type dressing, topped with 3 ounces fish or chicken

SNACK 3 *(ABF)*

Choose one of the following or an animal-based snack from chapter 10:

- 3 ounces cooked fresh crab
- ½ cup canned crab
- 4 cooked large sea scallops
- ½ cup low-fat cottage cheese with ¼ cup fresh pineapple slices

DAY 3

MEAL I

Choose one of the following:

- Blueberry toast: Spread 1 slice 100 percent whole-grain or 100 percent whole-wheat toast with 1 tablespoon blueberry jam, top with fresh blueberries and 1 slice cheese, and drizzle with ½ teaspoon honey.
- Banana toast: Spread 1 slice 100 percent whole-grain or 100 percent whole-wheat toast with a nut butter, then cover with thinly sliced bananas.
- Vegan bran muffin (or another muffin flavor) and 1 serving of fruit

SNACK I

Choose one of the following or a plant-based snack from chapter 10:

- 4 dried apricots with 15 dry-roasted almonds
- Organic nut or protein bar (150 calories or less)
- ¾ cup roasted chickpeas
- Kale bruschetta: Toast 1 slice 100 percent whole-grain or 100 percent whole-wheat bread, top with cooked kale leaves and halved grape tomatoes, season with salt and pepper to taste, and drizzle with balsamic vinaigrette.
- Small baked potato (white or sweet) topped with 2 tablespoons hummus

MEAL 2

Choose one of the following:

- Beets and Greens with Hazelnuts and Yogurt-Dill Sauce (see recipe on page 162)
- 1½ cups butternut squash, cucumber, chickpea, or black bean soup with ¾ cup brown rice
- Vegetable burrito bowl: Combine 2 cups brown rice, 1 cup beans of your choice, ½ small avocado, sliced, ⅓ cup shredded lettuce, and 2 tablespoons diced onion.

THREE DISEASE-FIGHTING PLANTS

Asparagus: These long green spears contain glutathione, a detoxifying compound that can remove harmful compounds such as carcinogens and free radicals from the body. Another benefit is that it has anti-inflammatory properties that help fight against several chronic diseases, such as type 2 diabetes and heart disease.

RED CABBAGE MICROGREENS: These purplish sprouts contain significant quantities of vitamins C and K. Vitamin C is a super antioxidant that fights inflammation and protects against cell damage.

BROCCOLI SPROUTS: Loaded with the compound sulforaphane, these tiny plants do a mighty job of mobilizing the body's natural cancer-fighting resources to help hinder tumor growth. These sprouts have also been shown to help protect the heart by lowering blood sugar and cholesterol levels. Sprouts are ten to thirty times more potent than fully grown broccoli.

SNACK 2

Choose one of the following or a plant-based snack from chapter 10:

- Dehydrated cinnamon apples: Thinly slice 3 medium apples. Sprinkle with cinnamon. Spread evenly on parchment paper in a baking dish. Place in a 170-degree oven for 5 to 6 hours, turning the slices every hour until browned and crispy. (Eat 1 apple's worth of slices as a snack and save the other two for later.)
- ½ red bell pepper, sliced, drizzled with balsamic vinaigrette and seasoned with salt and pepper
- Homemade sweet potato chips: Thinly slice 2 sweet potatoes and place in a bowl with 2 tablespoons olive oil and sea salt to taste. Place on an aluminum foil–lined baking sheet and bake in a 375-degree oven for 25 to 30 minutes until desired crispness. (Eat 1 cup of chips and save the rest for later.)
- Mediterranean salad: Dice 1 tomato, 1 small cucumber, and ¼ red onion. Drizzle with balsamic vinaigrette.
- ½ cup nut-free trail mix with no added sugar

MEAL 3

Choose one of the following:

- Creamy Vegan Penne with Asparagus, Edamame, and Mint (see recipe on page 174)
- Large salad (all or any of the following: ½ cup beans, 3 cups lettuce or other greens, 5 olives, 3 tablespoons shredded cheese, 5 cherry tomatoes, 2 tablespoons nuts,

sliced cucumbers) with 2 tablespoons low-fat or fat-free vinaigrette-type dressing

- 2 cups lentil soup with ¾ cup brown or white rice

SNACK 3

Choose one of the following or a plant-based snack from chapter 10:

- 1½ cups fresh fruit salad
- Black bean salsa over 3 roasted eggplant slices
- 1 cup miso soup
- 1 cup roasted or grilled zucchini slices seasoned with salt and/or pepper
- 1 tablespoon peanuts and 2 tablespoons dried cranberries

DAY 4

MEAL I (ABF)

Choose one of the following:
- 1½ cups cooked oatmeal or grits with berries or banana
- 2 scrambled eggs (cheese and vegetables optional) and 1 piece of fruit
- Bacon grilled cheese sandwich: Butter 1 side of 2 pieces of 100 percent whole-grain or 100 percent whole-wheat bread, then set aside. Cook 3 slices turkey or pork bacon. Place 1 piece of bread, buttered side down, in a skillet over medium heat. Place 1 piece of cheese on top of the bread, then cut the bacon strips in half and place on top of the cheese. Place a second piece of cheese on top of the bacon, then put the second piece of bread on top to complete the sandwich. Make sure the buttered side is facing up. Cook until golden brown and the cheese is melting, then flip and cook the second side.

SNACK I

Choose one of the following or a plant-based snack from chapter 10:
- 50 Goldfish crackers
- ½ cup kale chips
- ⅓ cup low-fat granola
- 3 cups air-popped popcorn
- 3 tablespoons roasted pumpkin seeds

MEAL 2 *(ABF)*

Choose one of the following:

- 1½ cups chicken and rice soup with a small green garden salad
- Avocado bacon salad: Chop half a head of romaine lettuce or 2 cups kale, and place in a bowl. Add ½ cup chopped cucumbers, ¼ cup chopped onions, and ½ avocado, sliced. Add 2 slices pork or turkey bacon, diced, then drizzle with 2 tablespoons of your choice of dressing.
- Cucumber tuna salad: Drain 1 can of tuna, then place in a bowl and mix in ½ cup peeled and diced cucumber, ½ tablespoon fresh lemon juice, 1 tablespoon mayonnaise, and a pinch of salt. Serve on a bed of greens or inside a whole-wheat tortilla.

SNACK 2

Choose one of the following or a plant-based snack from chapter 10:

- 40 shelled pistachios
- ¾ cup melon cubes
- 1 slice 100 percent whole-grain bread or 1 whole-wheat pita pocket, cut into quarters, with 2 tablespoons hummus
- 1 large apple, orange, or banana
- 10 baby carrots dipped in 2 tablespoons light salad dressing

MEAL 3 *(ABF)*

Choose one of the following:
- 6 ounces steamed scallops and 2 servings of vegetables
- Chicken stir-fry: Cook 6-ounce chicken breast, dice, then set aside. Add ¼ cup diced red bell peppers, ¼ cup diced tomatoes, 1 tablespoon diced onion, 1 teaspoon minced garlic, and a pinch each of salt and pepper to the skillet. Cook the vegetables for about 5 minutes, stirring frequently. Return the chicken and cook for another couple of minutes until heated through.
- 2 cups soup of your choice

SNACK 3

Choose one of the following or a plant-based snack from chapter 10:
- ¾ cup roasted chickpeas
- ¾ cup roasted black beans
- 3 hummus-and-veggie roll-ups
- 4 almond butter–stuffed dates
- 2 tablespoons refried bean dip (made without lard) and 5 tortilla chips

DAY 5

MEAL I

Choose one of the following:
- 3 to 4 servings of fruit
- 1 fruit smoothie (300 calories or less, no added sugars)
- 1½ cups whole-grain cereal with berries and 1 cup oat, soy, or almond milk

SNACK I *(ABF)*

Choose one of the following or an animal-based snack from chapter 10:
- Tomato-mozzarella salad: Cube 1 ounce fresh mozzarella and combine in small bowl with 11 halved cherry tomatoes and 2 teaspoons fresh chopped basil, then drizzle with 1 tablespoon balsamic vinaigrette
- 2 tablespoons hummus with 5 baby carrots
- 2 tablespoons hummus with ½ small cucumber, sliced
- Hot quesadilla: Spray 1 side of a corn tortilla with cooking spray, then place in a skillet over medium heat. Top with ¼ cup Mexican cheese blend, fold in half, and cook for a couple of minutes on each side until the cheese melts and the tortilla is slightly crisp. Serve with 2 tablespoons pico de gallo or salsa if desired.
- 1 cup 2 percent ultra-filtered chocolate milk

MEAL 2

Choose one of the following:

- Oven-Braised Fennel with Orange-Pecan Gremolata (see recipe on page 164)
- 1½ cups minestrone, onion, tomato, or carrot soup and ¾ cup brown rice
- Large salad (all or any of the following: ½ cup beans, 3 cups lettuce or other greens, 5 olives, 3 tablespoons shredded cheese, 5 cherry tomatoes, 2 tablespoons nuts, sliced cucumbers) with 2 tablespoons low-fat or fat-free vinaigrette-type dressing

MORE MILK THAN YOU THINK

It takes 21 pounds of milk to make 1 pound of butter.
It takes 12 pounds of milk to make 1 gallon of ice cream.
It takes 10 pounds of milk to make 1 pound of cheese.

SNACK 2

Choose one of the following or a plant-based snack from chapter 10:

- Small baked potato topped with salsa
- ¾ cup roasted cauliflower with a pinch of sea salt
- 1 cup blueberries with a dollop of whipped cream
- ½ large cucumber, cut in sticks or coins, dipped in 2 tablespoons hummus
- 6 dates

MEAL 3 *(ABF)*

Choose one of the following:

- 2 lobster tails with melted butter sauce and 2 servings of vegetables
- Spinach turkey salad: In a bowl, mix 2 cups baby spinach, ⅓ cup mushrooms, 1 chopped hard-boiled egg, 2 tablespoons chopped red onion, ¼ cup pecan or walnut halves, 1 teaspoon minced garlic, and ¼ cup dried cranberries, then top with 4 ounces turkey.
- 6-ounce steak, chicken, or fish with 2 servings of vegetables

SNACK 3

Choose one of the following or a plant-based snack from chapter 10:

- 1½ cups vegan chili topped with avocado slices
- ¾ cup roasted chickpeas
- ¾ cup roasted black beans
- ½ medium avocado sprinkled with a little squeeze of lime juice and sea salt
- 1 medium red bell pepper, sliced, with ¼ cup guacamole

DAY 6

MEAL 1 *(ABF)*

Choose one of the following:

- 2 slices french toast made with 100 percent whole-grain or 100 percent whole-wheat bread and ½ cup berries
- 8 ounces yogurt topped with berries and ¼ cup granola
- Omelet made with 2 eggs, cheese, and vegetables

SNACK 1

Choose one of the following or a plant-based snack from chapter 10:

- 5 pitted dates stuffed with 5 whole almonds
- ½ cup unsweetened applesauce mixed with 10 pecan halves
- ¼ cup low-fat granola
- 1 cup lettuce, drizzled with 2 tablespoons fat-free dressing
- 3 oven-baked potato wedges

MEAL 2 *(ABF)*

Choose one of the following:

- Chicken caprese salad: In a large bowl, toss 2 cups greens of your choice, ¾ cup diced chicken, ½ cup mozzarella (or cheese of your choice), ½ cup diced tomato, ¼ cup chopped fresh basil, 1 teaspoon extra-virgin olive oil, and 2 tablespoons fresh lemon juice.

- Power salmon bowl: In a bowl, place 2 cups chopped greens of your choice, 3 ounces of cooked salmon, chopped, ½ cup diced cucumbers, ¼ cup shredded carrots, ½ cup diced tomatoes, and ½ cup cooked brown rice. Drizzle with balsamic vinaigrette.
- Turkey or chicken club sandwich on 100 percent whole-grain or 100 percent whole-wheat bread with lettuce, tomato, cheese, and 2 teaspoons condiments of your choice.

SNACK 2

Choose one of the following or a plant-based snack from chapter 10:

- 2 frozen fruit bars (no sugar added)
- 2 tablespoons hummus spread on 4 crackers
- 10 black olives
- ½ cup quinoa or brown rice
- 5 baby carrots and 3 tablespoons hummus

MEAL 3 (ABF)

Choose one of the following:

- 3 giant crab legs with melted butter sauce and 2 servings of vegetables
- 1 piece of meat lasagna (4 inches × 3 inches × 2 inches) with 2 servings of vegetables
- 2 cups chicken or beef stir-fry

SNACK 3

Choose one of the following or a plant-based snack from chapter 10:

- 2 cups grilled or roasted broccoli florets
- 17 pecans
- 25 cherries
- 6 dried apricots
- 1 rice cake with 1 tablespoon guacamole

DAY 7

MEAL I

Choose one of the following:

- 1 protein shake (300 calories or less, no added sugars)
- 1½ cups cold or hot cereal with 1 cup almond, coconut, or soy milk
- ½ avocado, mashed and spread on 2 pieces of 100 percent whole-grain or 100 percent whole-wheat toast

SNACK I

Choose one of the following or a plant-based snack from chapter 10:

- 2 dill pickle spears
- 2 frozen fruit bars (no sugar added)
- ½ cup wasabi peas
- ½ cup raw or cooked vegetables
- 12 baked tortilla chips and ½ cup salsa

MEAL 2

Choose one of the following:

- Cabbage Steaks with Marinated White Bean Couscous (see recipe on page 166)
- 1½ cups vegetable, white bean, or miso soup with ¾ cup brown rice
- 1½ cups whole-wheat pasta mixed with vegetables of your choice

YOU GET OUT WHAT YOU PUT IN

Not all plant-based diets are created equal. It's possible to consume plant-based foods that are of low quality and have little or no nutritional or health benefits. You need to make sure you focus on eating as cleanly as possible and reducing the number of processed ingredients and amount of added sugars and unhealthy fats. Eating a quality plant-based diet can lower your risk of dying from heart disease by as much as 25 percent; however, consuming an unhealthy one can actually *increase* your risk by 32 percent. Research has also indicated that improving the quality of a plant-based diet over twelve years might reduce the likelihood of premature death by 10 percent. However, reducing the quality of your plant-based diet over the same period of time may increase your risk of premature death by 12 percent.

SNACK 2

Choose one of the following or a plant-based snack from chapter 10:

- Small baked potato topped with 2 tablespoons salsa
- 1 kiwi, sliced, with ½ cup oat cereal
- 6 dried figs
- 1½ cups diced watermelon
- 1 cup grape tomatoes, halved and sprinkled with sea salt

MEAL 3

Choose one of the following:

- Spicy Collard-Stuffed Sweet Potatoes (see recipe on page 171)
- 4 servings of roasted vegetables
- 1 piece of vegetable lasagna (4 inches × 3 inches × 2 inches)

SNACK 3

Choose one of the following or a plant-based snack from chapter 10:

- 1 cup sugar snap peas with 3 tablespoons hummus
- 5 pieces of brown rice vegetable sushi rolls
- 20 grapes with 15 peanuts
- 20 almonds
- 1 baked sweet potato with 1 teaspoon butter

Congratulations on your dietary and mental transformation! In these last four weeks, you've accomplished what often takes several years. If it hasn't become apparent to you yet, you will learn how much easier it is to find new and exciting dishes as a plant-based eater. Your newfound flexibility will allow you to eat at a broad array of restaurants, and there will rarely be a time when you can't find something appealing on a menu.

Being a plant-based eater does not mean you won't enjoy beef, chicken, or fish, but it does mean you can go long stretches without meat and not be upset about it. In fact, many people not only lose their taste preference for meat, they also feel like fatty meat is now too thick and sludge-like compared to plant-based foods. When you sit down to a meal full of plant-based foods, think about not just how great the fuel is you're putting into your body but also the positive impact that one meal has on helping to sustain and protect our planet so that generations yet to come can enjoy the bountiful opportunities this world has to offer. Make sure you allow yourself to be creative in your food choices and open your mind to varied exciting recipes from around the world full of wonderful flavors and nutritional benefits. Keep up the quality of the foods you eat, making sure they come from the best sources and have been processed as little as possible.

Hopefully, now that you've completed the four-week Plant Power program, you won't need to continue to rigorously follow the meal plan but can instead make instinctive choices that gratify your new palate. If you need to lose weight, challenge yourself to not only abide by the new 70:30 rule of plant-based to animal-based but also add regular exercise to your regimen (thirty minutes four to five days per week and mix cardio with resistance training) and even try some intermittent fasting. There's no doubt that a predominantly plant-based diet can deliver a multitude of life-changing benefits; it's just a matter of how much you embrace the possibilities and commit yourself to the journey. Eat well, live well!

9

PLANT
POWER
RECIPES

ARTICHOKE AND CHICKPEA CAESAR SALAD

SERVES 4

One 14-ounce can chickpeas, rinsed and drained

¼ cup extra-virgin olive oil, divided

1 tablespoon cornstarch

Kosher salt and freshly ground black pepper

½ teaspoon ground cumin

½ teaspoon ground coriander

Pinch cayenne pepper, optional

3 tablespoons fresh lemon juice

1 teaspoon dijon mustard

⅓ cup finely grated parmesan cheese, plus more for serving

One 14-ounce can quartered artichoke hearts in water, drained

3 romaine hearts, coarsely chopped

Preheat the oven to 425°F and line a baking sheet with aluminum foil.

Put the chickpeas in a mixing bowl and toss them with 1 teaspoon of the oil. In a small bowl, stir together the cornstarch, ½ teaspoon salt, ¼ teaspoon pepper, cumin, coriander, and cayenne , if using, and sprinkle it over the chickpeas. Using a large rubber spatula, toss the chickpeas until evenly coated in the spice mix. Evenly spread them on the lined baking sheet and roast in the oven, shaking the baking sheet occasionally to toss them, until they turn golden and crisp, 10 to 12 minutes. Transfer to a paper towel–lined plate to cool.

In a large mixing bowl, whisk the remaining oil, lemon juice, mustard, and ½ teaspoon each salt and pepper until combined; add the cheese and whisk to combine. Add the artichokes to the bowl and toss with a rubber spatula until evenly coated; add the lettuce and toss until well dressed. Transfer the salad to a serving platter. Scatter the chickpeas over the top and serve with additional parmesan cheese at the table.

CRISPY SALMON BURGERS

SERVES 4

---

1 pound salmon, coarsely diced

¼ cup chopped fresh flat-leaf parsley

3 tablespoons bread crumbs

1½ tablespoons finely diced red onion

2 cloves garlic, minced

½ teaspoon salt

¼ teaspoon freshly ground black pepper

1 tablespoon fresh lime juice

2 tablespoons extra-virgin olive oil

4 whole-wheat buns

Combine the salmon, parsley, bread crumbs, onion, garlic, salt, pepper, and lime juice in a blender. Blend on high for 2 minutes, scraping down the sides of the blender as necessary.

Remove the mixture from the blender and form 4 equal patties.

Heat the olive oil in a large sauté pan over medium-high heat. Sear the patties for about 4 minutes on each side, or until the outside is seared and the patties are cooked to medium doneness (or to desired doneness).

Transfer the patties to a clean plate. Toast the buns top-side down in the pan. Serve the patties on the warm, toasted buns.

ARUGULA SALAD
WITH ROASTED NEW POTATOES
AND PICKLED PEPPER DRESSING

SERVES 4

12 ounces multicolored baby potatoes, unpeeled, halved

¼ cup extra-virgin olive oil, divided

½ teaspoon dried thyme

Kosher salt and freshly ground black pepper

¼ cup pickled sweet peppers (Peppadews), drained, plus 3 tablespoons liquid from the jar

1 tablespoon whole-grain mustard

⅓ cup fresh basil leaves, minced

5 ounces baby arugula

One 2-ounce piece aged Gouda cheese

Preheat the oven to 450°F. Spread the potatoes on a baking sheet and drizzle 2 tablespoons of the oil over them; add the dried thyme, season with salt and pepper, and toss to coat. Roast in the oven, stirring halfway through, until golden brown and cooked through, 35 to 40 minutes.

Meanwhile, finely mince the peppers and put them in a large bowl. Add the liquid from the jar, the remaining olive oil, mustard, and basil and whisk until combined. When the potatoes are cooked, add them hot to the bowl of dressing and toss to coat. Let stand for 10 minutes to cool.

Add the arugula to the bowl and toss gently until evenly dressed. Transfer the salad to a serving platter; using a vegetable peeler, shave the cheese over the top of the salad and serve.

BARLEY WITH CRISPY BRUSSELS SPROUTS, WHITE BEANS, AND BROWNED BUTTER VINAIGRETTE

SERVES 4

1 pound brussels sprouts

2 tablespoons extra-virgin olive oil

Kosher salt and freshly ground black pepper

½ teaspoon ground cumin

½ teaspoon ground coriander

12 ounces pearl barley

One 14-ounce can cannellini beans, drained but not rinsed

3 tablespoons unsalted butter

1 teaspoon whole-grain dijon mustard

¼ cup cider vinegar

1 teaspoon chopped fresh thyme

Preheat the oven to 425°F.

Halve the brussels sprouts lengthwise, then cut the cores off each half so that most of the leaves fall away from the core. In a large bowl, whisk the oil, ½ teaspoon each salt and pepper, cumin, and coriander until combined. Add the brussels sprouts and toss well to coat. Transfer to a baking sheet and roast, stirring occasionally, until the edges are crisp and browned, about 20 minutes. Remove from the oven and let cool slightly.

Meanwhile, bring a large pot of water to a boil, add 1 teaspoon salt, and stir in the barley. Simmer, stirring frequently, until cooked through according to the package instructions. Drain and transfer to a mixing bowl. Stir in the beans and let stand until heated through.

Over medium heat, melt the butter in a medium saucepan; continue cooking, swirling the butter in the pan, until the butter begins to turn golden brown and smells nutty, 3 to 4 minutes. Remove from the heat and whisk in the mustard and vinegar until well combined; add ½ teaspoon salt, ¼ teaspoon pepper, and the thyme leaves and whisk until combined. Pour the warm dressing over the barley and beans, add the brussels sprouts, and toss well until evenly combined and dressed. Serve warm.

ENERGY BLAST YOGURT

The best breakfast to start the day includes fresh, eye-opening flavors that will get you up and moving without making you feel full or setting you up for a midmorning crash. Combining the staying power of oats, a blast of sweetness from fruit and honey, and the pleasing smoothness of yogurt, this one-bowl treat will get you off on the right foot. You can even count on a big helping of antioxidants from those mouth-watering blueberries!

SERVES 1

⅔ cup plain nonfat Greek yogurt

½ teaspoon honey

Pinch ground cinnamon

2 tablespoons rolled oats

Finely grated zest of 1 lemon

1 tablespoon dried blueberries

1 teaspoon roasted unsalted sunflower seeds

In a small bowl, combine the yogurt, honey, cinnamon, oats, and lemon zest and stir to mix. Let stand about 5 minutes to soften the oats. Sprinkle the blueberries and sunflower seeds over the top and enjoy.

BEETS AND GREENS WITH HAZELNUTS AND YOGURT-DILL SAUCE

SERVES 4

1½ pounds large red beets, peeled and cut into
1-inch chunks

2 cloves garlic, smashed

1 small bay leaf

1 bunch red chard, leaves stripped, stems reserved
and chopped, and leaves roughly chopped

Kosher salt and freshly ground black pepper

¾ cup low-fat yogurt, dairy or vegan

4 scallions, very finely chopped

½ cup finely chopped dill leaves, divided

½ teaspoon ground cumin

⅓ cup skinned hazelnuts, toasted

Put the beets, garlic, and bay leaf in a large saucepan, fill it with water, and bring it to a boil over high heat. Reduce the heat to medium and cook until the beets are just tender when pierced with a knife, 35 to 40 minutes. Add the chopped chard stems and cook for 3 minutes; stir in the chard leaves and cook until wilted but not mushy, 1 to 2 minutes. Drain the vegetables in a colander and toss them with ½ teaspoon each salt and pepper. Drain well, shaking the colander to remove all moisture, and transfer them to a serving platter. Remove the garlic and bay leaf.

Meanwhile, in a medium bowl, stir together the yogurt,

scallions, all but 2 tablespoons of the dill, cumin, ½ teaspoon salt, and ¼ teaspoon black pepper until combined.

To serve, drizzle some of the yogurt sauce over the beets and greens, and pass the rest at the table. Garnish with the hazelnuts and remaining dill.

OVEN-BRAISED FENNEL WITH ORANGE-PECAN GREMOLATA

SERVES 4

2 large fennel bulbs, trimmed, fronds reserved

4 sprigs fresh thyme

Extra-virgin olive oil

Kosher salt and freshly ground black pepper, plus 1 teaspoon peppercorns

3 cloves garlic, smashed, divided

1 bay leaf

2 cups vegetable broth

1 navel orange

¼ cup pecans, toasted

½ cup fresh flat-leaf parsley leaves

Preheat the oven to 350°F and position a rack in the center.

Halve each fennel bulb through the core and carefully slice each half into 4 wedges, being sure to cut through the core and keep the wedge intact. Arrange the thyme sprigs in a 9×13-inch baking dish and position the fennel wedges on top of them in a single layer. Brush the wedges with olive oil and season with salt and pepper. Add 2 of the garlic cloves and the bay leaf to the dish; pour the vegetable broth into the dish, cover with foil, and roast in the oven until the fennel is tender when pierced with a knife in the thickest part, about 1 hour. Uncover the dish, return it to the oven, and raise the temperature to 425°F. Continue cooking until the fennel is golden brown and the liquid has mostly evaporated, about 15 minutes more.

Meanwhile, using a vegetable peeler, zest the orange in long, thin strips without removing any of the white pith. Transfer the orange peel to a food processor, add the pecans and remaining garlic clove, and pulse until finely chopped. Add the parsley leaves, fennel fronds, ½ teaspoon salt, and ¼ teaspoon pepper and pulse until finely chopped but not pulverized. Transfer to a bowl.

With a slotted spoon, transfer the fennel to a serving platter, leaving the thyme and bay leaf in the baking dish. Spoon a little of any liquid left in the dish over the fennel. Spoon a little of the orange gremolata over each fennel wedge and serve the remainder at the table.

CABBAGE STEAKS WITH MARINATED WHITE BEAN COUSCOUS

SERVES 4

---

1 large head savoy cabbage, trimmed

Extra-virgin olive oil

Kosher salt and freshly ground black pepper

1¼ cups vegetable broth or water

1 cup multicolored couscous

2 tablespoons cider vinegar

1 teaspoon dried Italian seasoning

Pinch red chili flakes

One 15-ounce can cannellini beans, drained

½ cup fresh flat-leaf parsley leaves, finely chopped, divided

2 plum tomatoes, cored, seeded, and finely chopped

Preheat the oven to 400°F. Line a baking sheet with aluminum foil.

Stand the cabbage upright on its core, and using a sharp knife, carefully slice the cabbage from top to bottom into 4 equal slices, about 1 inch thick. Transfer the slices to the baking sheet, maintaining enough distance between them so they're not touching. Brush the surface with about 1 tablespoon olive oil; season well with salt and pepper. Roast in the oven, rotating the sheet halfway through, until the core is soft and the outer leaves are browned and crisp, 40 to 45 minutes. Remove from the oven and transfer the slices to a serving platter.

Meanwhile, bring the vegetable broth and ½ teaspoon salt to a simmer in a small saucepan over medium heat; stir in the couscous, cover, and remove from the heat.

In a medium bowl, whisk 3 tablespoons olive oil, the vinegar, Italian seasoning, chili flakes, and ¼ teaspoon salt together until combined. Add the beans and toss gently until evenly dressed.

Fluff the couscous with a fork and transfer it to the bowl with the beans along with ¾ of the parsley. Toss gently until well combined and evenly dressed; taste and season with salt and pepper.

Spoon the bean and couscous salad over the cabbage steaks; garnish with the remaining parsley and the diced tomatoes. Drizzle with additional olive oil, if desired, and serve.

CITRUS-MASALA KALE CHIPS

SERVES 4

---

1 tablespoon grapeseed or sunflower oil

Finely grated zest of ½ lemon

Finely grated zest of ½ lime

1¼ teaspoons garam masala spice OR ½ teaspoon ground cumin, ¼ teaspoon ground coriander, ¼ teaspoon ground cardamom, ¼ teaspoon ground cinnamon, pinch black pepper, and pinch ground cloves

1 bunch kale, about 1 pound, washed, patted dry, and stems removed

Kosher salt

Preheat the oven to 250°F. Line a baking sheet with parchment paper.

In a large bowl, whisk together the oil, lemon and lime zests, and garam masala until combined. Add the kale, and using a rubber spatula, toss the kale, pressing on it with the spatula to fully coat the leaves with the spice mixture. Spread the leaves in an even layer on the baking sheet and lightly sprinkle with salt. Bake in the oven, stirring once, until very crisp and beginning to turn light golden brown, about 45 minutes.

Cool completely on the baking sheet. Serve as a snack, and store any leftovers in an airtight bag at room temperature.

TOMATO AND WHITE BEAN SOUP

SERVES 4 (MAKES ABOUT 6 CUPS)

1 tablespoon extra-virgin olive oil

1 yellow onion, chopped

2 cloves garlic, minced

1 teaspoon tomato paste

1 large sprig fresh thyme

1 small bay leaf

Kosher salt and freshly ground black pepper

One 15-ounce can diced tomatoes, with liquid

One 15-ounce can white beans (cannellini or navy), drained

1 quart low-sodium chicken stock (or substitute low-sodium vegetable broth)

Heat the olive oil in a large saucepan over medium-high heat. Add the onion and garlic and cook until softened, about 4 minutes. Add the tomato paste and cook, stirring, until the paste begins to caramelize, 2 to 3 minutes.

Add the thyme, bay leaf, salt, and pepper. Add the tomatoes and liquid and bring the mixture to a boil. Cook until most of the liquid evaporates, about 5 minutes.

Add the beans and chicken stock and cook until the beans begin to break down, about 10 minutes.

Remove the bay leaf and thyme sprig. Carefully transfer about 1 cup of the soup to a food processor, purée, and return the mixture to the saucepan (or use a handheld immersion mixer to purée about ¼ of the soup in the saucepan, until it has thickened).

Season with salt and pepper to taste. Serve warm.

SPICY COLLARD-STUFFED SWEET POTATOES

SERVES 4

Cooking spray

3 tablespoons olive oil, divided

2 large sweet potatoes, halved lengthwise

Kosher salt and freshly ground black pepper

2 large shallots, sliced

2 cloves garlic, minced

2 fresno chilies, seeded and chopped

1 bunch, about 12 ounces, collard greens, stems removed, coarsely chopped

1 teaspoon smoked paprika, plus more for serving

Preheat the oven to 400°F. Line a baking sheet with aluminum foil and spray it with cooking spray. Brush 1 tablespoon of the oil over the surface of the potatoes and season them generously with salt and pepper. Roast them, cut sides down, until a knife inserted in them meets no resistance, about 40 minutes. Transfer them upright to a platter and cool briefly.

Heat the remaining oil in a large pot over medium-high heat; add the shallots and cook, stirring, until softened and beginning to brown, 3 to 4 minutes. Add the garlic and chilies and cook, stirring, until softened, 1 to 2 minutes. Add the collard greens, paprika, 1 teaspoon salt, ½ teaspoon pepper, and ½ cup water; toss with tongs until the leaves begin to soften. Cover, reduce the heat to medium, and cook, tossing occasionally, until the greens are completely soft but not mushy, about 45 minutes. Taste and adjust seasoning with salt and pepper.

Using a sharp knife, score the potatoes without cutting through the skins and break up the flesh with a fork. Top each potato half with ¼ of the greens, sprinkle with paprika, and serve.

SERIOUSLY SIMPLE CHICKEN SALAD

SERVES 4

2 cups chopped cooked skinless, boneless chicken breast

1 stalk celery, cut in half

½ avocado, chopped

½ red bell pepper, chopped

½ cup low-fat herb vinaigrette

¼ cup chopped fresh cilantro

2 scallions, trimmed and cut in half

4 whole-wheat buns

4 slices tomato

Combine the chicken, celery, avocado, pepper, vinaigrette, cilantro, and scallions in a blender. Pulse until the texture is coarse and the mixture is well blended.

Divide the salad among the four buns, top each with a slice of tomato, and serve.

CREAMY VEGAN PENNE WITH ASPARAGUS, EDAMAME, AND MINT

SERVES 4

1 cup dairy-free sour cream

Kosher salt and freshly ground black pepper

1 teaspoon finely grated lemon zest

½ teaspoon finely grated fresh garlic

1 pound whole-grain penne

8 ounces asparagus, trimmed and cut into 1-inch pieces

½ cup shelled frozen edamame, thawed

⅓ cup loosely packed fresh mint leaves, thinly sliced, divided

Grated vegan parmesan cheese, for serving, optional

In a small bowl, stir together the sour cream, ½ teaspoon salt, ¼ teaspoon pepper, lemon zest, and garlic until combined. Set aside.

Bring 2 quarts of water and 1 tablespoon salt to a boil in a large pot; stir in the pasta and cook for 10 minutes. Remove ½ cup of the cooking water, stir in the asparagus, and cook until the asparagus is tender and the pasta is al dente, about 2 minutes more. Drain the pasta and return to the pot.

Return the pot with the pasta to medium heat, add the reserved cooking water and the edamame, and simmer, stirring, until the water is absorbed, 1 to 2 minutes. Remove from the heat and stir in the sour cream mixture; let stand until heated through. Taste and adjust seasoning with salt and pepper; stir in half of the mint until combined and transfer the pasta to a serving bowl. Scatter the remaining mint over the top and serve with parmesan cheese, if using.

SMOKED SALMON AND EGG SANDWICH

SERVES 4

¼ cup fat-free cream cheese, at room temperature

1 teaspoon capers, drained

½ teaspoon dried dill

4 whole-wheat english muffins, split and toasted

Cooking spray

4 large eggs

Kosher salt and freshly ground black pepper

4 ounces smoked salmon (no added sugar)

In a small bowl, mash the cream cheese with a rubber spatula until very smooth and spreadable. Add the capers and dill and stir well to combine. Spread about 1 tablespoon of the mixture on the bottom half of each muffin.

Coat a large nonstick skillet with cooking spray and heat it over medium heat. Cook the eggs sunny-side up. Season with salt and pepper to taste and cook to desired doneness.

Set 1 egg on each cream cheese–covered muffin. Divide the salmon among the sandwiches, cover with the muffin tops, and serve.

CRISPY ZUCCHINI FINGERS WITH GREEN GODDESS DIP

SERVES 4

3 medium zucchini, about 1½ pounds total, stemmed

1 cup whole-wheat panko bread crumbs

½ teaspoon dried thyme

Kosher salt and freshly ground black pepper

½ cup cornstarch

1 cup soy or almond milk

2 ripe avocados, peeled, pitted, and roughly chopped

3 scallions, chopped

⅓ cup fresh parsley leaves

¼ cup fat-free plain yogurt (Greek, soy, or other vegan)

3 tablespoons rice vinegar

Preheat the oven to 400°F. Line a baking sheet with parchment.

Halve the zucchini lengthwise and then cut them in half crosswise. Depending on how thick they are, cut the halves into ½- to 1-inch wedges. On a large plate, stir together the bread crumbs, thyme, and ½ teaspoon each salt and pepper. Put the cornstarch on a shallow plate and the milk into a shallow bowl.

Working a few at a time, dredge the zucchini wedges with cornstarch, shaking off the excess, then dip each wedge in the milk until just coated and lay them on the bread crumbs. Coat the zucchini all over in bread crumbs, pressing lightly to adhere, and transfer them to the baking sheet. Bake, turning once halfway through, until golden brown and the zucchini is tender but still holds its shape, 20 to 25 minutes. Cool briefly on the baking sheet.

Meanwhile, put the avocado, scallions, parsley, yogurt, rice vinegar, ½ teaspoon salt, and ¼ teaspoon pepper in a food processor and purée until smooth. Taste and adjust seasoning if needed. If the dressing is very thick, add water, a few tablespoons at a time, until it is the consistency of thin sour cream.

Transfer the zucchini wedges to a platter and serve with the Green Goddess dressing for dipping.

CHICKEN AND MUSHROOM STIR-FRY

SERVES 4

3 teaspoons canola oil, divided

3 large shallots, sliced lengthwise

6 ounces cremini mushrooms, quartered

6 ounces shiitake mushrooms, sliced

2 large cloves garlic, chopped

1 teaspoon peeled and finely chopped fresh ginger

12 ounces chicken tenders, cut into 1-inch pieces

2 teaspoons reduced-sodium soy sauce

1 teaspoon rice vinegar

½ teaspoon toasted sesame oil

1 teaspoon cornstarch

4 scallions, chopped

Heat 1 teaspoon of the canola oil in a wok or large non-stick skillet over medium-high heat. Swirl the pan until the oil is very hot. Add the shallots and mushrooms and stir-fry, stirring constantly, until the shallots are softened and the mushrooms release their liquid and begin to brown (6 to 8 minutes). Add the garlic and ginger and cook, stirring, for about 2 minutes more. Transfer the vegetables to a bowl and set aside.

Add the remaining 2 teaspoons of canola oil to the wok and heat. Add the chicken and stir-fry until cooked and no pink remains, about 5 minutes. Return the mushroom mixture to the wok and stir to combine.

In a small bowl, combine the soy sauce, rice vinegar, sesame oil, and cornstarch and stir until smooth. Pour this mixture into the wok and cook, stirring, until the liquid begins to bubble and thicken. It should glaze the chicken and vegetables.

Add the scallions and toss several times. Remove to a serving bowl and serve immediately.

CUCUMBER, WATERMELON, AND AVOCADO SALAD WITH CHILI-MINT VINAIGRETTE

SERVES 4

½ english cucumber, halved lengthwise, seeded, and sliced

2 pounds watermelon, cubed, about 3 cups

¼ cup rice vinegar

2 teaspoons dijon mustard

⅓ cup sunflower or grapeseed oil

Kosher salt and freshly ground black pepper

1 fresno chili, stemmed, seeded, and minced

⅓ cup fresh mint leaves, finely chopped

2 avocados, peeled, pitted, and diced

¼ cup roasted, salted sunflower seeds

Put the cucumber and melon in a large bowl.

In a small bowl, whisk the vinegar and mustard together until combined. While whisking, slowly add the oil until emulsified; add ½ teaspoon salt and ¼ teaspoon pepper and mix well. Add the chili and mint to the dressing and stir to combine. Drizzle ¾ of the dressing over the cucumber and melon and gently toss with a rubber spatula until evenly dressed.

Transfer the cucumber mixture to a serving platter and scatter the avocado evenly over it. Spoon the remaining dressing over the salad, season with a little salt, sprinkle the sunflower seeds over the top, and serve.

SPICY CARROT AND CELERY ROOT SOUP

SERVES 4 (MAKES ABOUT 6 CUPS)

1 tablespoon extra-virgin olive oil

2 large shallots, chopped

2 cloves garlic, smashed

1 tablespoon peeled and grated fresh ginger

½ small jalapeño, seeded and chopped

3 large carrots, peeled and chopped

1 medium celery root, peeled and roughly chopped

½ cup orange juice

1 quart vegetable broth

Kosher salt and freshly ground black pepper

Juice of 1 lemon

4 scallions, sliced, for garnish

Heat the olive oil in a large saucepan over medium heat. Add the shallots and garlic and cook until softened, about 5 minutes. Add the ginger and jalapeño and stir well.

Add the carrots, celery root, and orange juice and bring to a simmer. Stir until the liquid has reduced slightly, 2 to 3 minutes.

Add the vegetable broth, season with salt and pepper, and bring the mixture to a boil. Reduce the heat to medium-low, cover, and cook until the carrots and celery root are completely soft and falling apart, 30 to 40 minutes.

Working in batches, purée the soup in a blender or with

a handheld immersion blender. Return the soup to the pan. Season with lemon juice, salt, and pepper to taste.

Ladle the soup into bowls, garnish with scallions, and serve warm.

FENNEL, CELERY ROOT, AND APPLE SALAD WITH PITA CROUTONS

SERVES 4

1 pita, split horizontally into 2 rounds

¼ cup grapeseed or sunflower oil, divided

1 teaspoon ground coriander, divided

Kosher salt

3 tablespoons cider vinegar

1 teaspoon honey

1 celery root, about 1 pound, peeled and cut into matchsticks

2 medium fennel bulbs, trimmed, fronds reserved, cored, and very thinly sliced

2 crisp red apples, such as Gala or Honeycrisp, cut into matchsticks

1 teaspoon whole-grain mustard

Freshly ground black pepper

1 tablespoon chopped fresh tarragon or 1 teaspoon dried

Preheat the oven to 400°F.

Put the pita halves on a baking sheet and brush them with 2 tablespoons of the oil. Sprinkle half the coriander on both sides along with salt to taste. Bake in the oven, turning once, until just golden but not too brown, 8 to 10 minutes. Set aside to cool.

In a medium bowl, whisk the vinegar and honey together until combined; add the celery root and toss to coat. Let stand for 15 minutes. Using a large slotted spoon, transfer the celery root to a serving bowl and add the fennel and apples to it.

To the bowl with the vinegar-honey mixture, whisk in the remaining coriander, mustard, ½ teaspoon salt, and ¼ teaspoon black pepper until combined. While whisking, slowly drizzle in the remaining oil until emulsified and the mixture is smooth. Drizzle the dressing over the vegetables and apples and toss to coat. Let stand for 10 minutes.

Add the tarragon to the salad, toss, taste, and season with additional salt and pepper. Break the crisp pita into large pieces over the top, garnish with the fennel fronds, and serve.

MEAT-STUFFED PEPPERS

SERVES 4

4 large red bell peppers (or use a combination of colors)
2 tablespoons olive oil, divided
1 pound lean ground beef
1 medium onion, chopped
2 cloves garlic, minced
2 tablespoons chili powder
1 teaspoon dried oregano
1 teaspoon brown mustard
½ teaspoon onion powder
Kosher salt and freshly ground black pepper
One-half 14.5-ounce can diced tomatoes
One 8-ounce can tomato sauce
¼ cup tomato paste
1 cup cooked brown or green lentils
3 tablespoons grated parmesan cheese

Position an oven rack 8 inches from the heat source and pre-heat the broiler. Line a roasting pan with aluminum foil.

Bring a large pot of water to boil over high heat. Cut the tops off the bell peppers and remove the seeds and membranes. Rinse the peppers under cold water.

Add the bell peppers to the pot, reduce the heat, and simmer for 5 minutes, or until tender. Drain and set the peppers aside.

In a large skillet over medium-high heat, heat 1 tablespoon of the olive oil. Brown the beef. Remove the beef with a slotted spoon and set aside.

Pour out the excess grease from the skillet and heat the skillet over medium-high heat. Add the remaining olive oil.

Add the onion and garlic. Stir until softened and fragrant, 2 to 3 minutes. Add the chili powder, oregano, mustard, and onion powder, and stir to coat the vegetables. Season with salt and pepper to taste.

Add the tomatoes, tomato sauce, and tomato paste. Stir to combine and simmer for 3 to 4 minutes. Add the meat and lentils and simmer until heated through.

Fill the bell peppers with the beef mixture and place them upright in the roasting pan. Top with the parmesan. Broil for 3 to 5 minutes, or until the parmesan is golden brown.

FUSILLI WITH GREEN BEANS, TOMATOES, AND TOASTED GARLIC

SERVES 4

Kosher salt

1 pound whole-grain fusilli

3 tablespoons extra-virgin olive oil

4 large cloves garlic, thinly sliced

8 ounces green beans, trimmed and cut into
1-inch pieces

2 shallots, minced

1 tablespoon tomato paste

1 pint multicolored cherry tomatoes, halved

Freshly ground black pepper

Bring a large pot of water to a boil and add 1 tablespoon salt; stir in the pasta and cook until just shy of al dente, according to the package instructions. Reserve 1 cup of the cooking water and drain. Return the pasta to the pot.

Meanwhile, stir the oil and garlic together in a large skillet over medium heat. Cook, stirring frequently, until the garlic begins to turn light golden brown, 3 to 4 minutes (do not overcook); using a slotted spoon, transfer the garlic to a paper towel–lined plate.

Raise the heat to medium-high, add the green beans, and cook, stirring only a couple of times, until the beans begin to char and are crisp-tender, 5 to 6 minutes. Using the slotted spoon, transfer the beans to the pot with the pasta. Return the skillet to medium-high, add the shallots, and cook, stirring, until softened, about 2 minutes. Add the tomato paste and cook, stirring, until the paste begins to brown, 2 to 3 minutes. Pour in the reserved pasta cooking water and cook, stirring, until the liquid simmers and the tomato paste dissolves and the broth thickens slightly, 2 to 3 minutes.

Pour the tomato-shallot broth into the pot with the pasta and beans and stir in the tomatoes. Set the pot over medium heat and cook, stirring gently, until the liquid simmers and is absorbed, and the tomatoes have softened, 4 to 5 minutes. Taste and season with salt and pepper.

Transfer to a serving bowl, top with the toasted garlic slices, and serve.

GRILLED ZUCCHINI AND EGGPLANT WITH SRIRACHA-SESAME VINAIGRETTE

SERVES 4

¼ cup grapeseed or sunflower oil, divided

2 teaspoons honey, divided

1 medium globe eggplant, about 1 pound, stemmed and cut lengthwise into 8 wedges

2 medium zucchini, about 1 pound total, quartered lengthwise

Kosher salt and freshly ground black pepper

¼ cup sriracha sauce or your favorite chili sauce

¼ cup rice vinegar

2 teaspoons toasted sesame oil

Toasted sesame seeds and torn fresh mint leaves, for serving

Preheat a gas grill or stovetop grill pan to medium-high. In a small bowl, whisk together 2 tablespoons of the oil and 1 teaspoon of the honey; brush the eggplant and zucchini all over with the mixture, and season the vegetables with salt and pepper. Place the eggplant spears cut side down on the grill or pan and cook without turning, until grill marks begin to appear, about 5 minutes; turn to the other cut side and grill until marks appear, 3 to 4 minutes. Flip the spears to the skin side and cook until the eggplant is softened but still holds its shape, 3 to 4 minutes longer. Transfer to a platter. Place the zucchini spears on the grill and cook, turning once, until lightly charred and softened but still holding their shape, 5 to 6 minutes; transfer to the platter with the eggplant.

In a medium bowl, whisk the remaining oil, remaining honey, sriracha, vinegar, sesame oil, and ½ teaspoon each salt and pepper until combined. Drizzle the dressing over the vegetables, sprinkle with sesame seeds and mint, and serve warm or at room temperature.

HASSELBACK POTATOES WITH SALSA VERDE

SERVES 4

> 4 large red potatoes, (about 12 ounces each), unpeeled, washed and dried
>
> 6 tablespoons avocado, grapeseed, or sunflower oil, divided
>
> 1 large clove garlic, smashed, plus 2 small cloves garlic
>
> ½ teaspoon ground cumin
>
> Kosher salt and freshly ground black pepper
>
> 1 cup fresh flat-leaf parsley leaves
>
> ½ cup fresh mint leaves
>
> ⅓ cup fresh dill leaves
>
> 1 small shallot, roughly chopped
>
> 2 tablespoons drained capers
>
> 2 teaspoons white wine vinegar

Preheat the oven to 350°F.

Halve the potatoes lengthwise. Place a potato half, cut side down, on a cutting board and position 2 chopsticks on each long side of the potato. Using a sharp knife, thinly slice the potato crosswise about every ⅛ inch, using the chopsticks as a guide to prevent cutting all the way through. Transfer the potato to a baking dish; repeat with the remaining potatoes.

In a small bowl, whisk 3 tablespoons of the avocado oil with the large garlic clove and cumin until combined. Brush the potatoes with ¾ of the mixture on all sides, being sure to brush the cut sides as well so they don't stick to the pan. Very lightly season the potatoes with salt and pepper. Roast for 1 hour, brushing the remaining oil mixture over the tops of the potatoes halfway through, until golden brown and tender.

Meanwhile, put the parsley, mint, dill, shallot, capers, and 2 small garlic cloves in a food processor and pulse until very finely chopped. Transfer to a bowl; stir in the remaining 3 tablespoons oil, vinegar, ¼ teaspoon salt, and a pinch of black pepper until combined. Taste and adjust seasoning.

Transfer the potatoes to a serving platter and spoon some of the salsa verde over the top of each; serve the rest at the table. These potatoes make a great side dish or a full meal with a sweet butter lettuce salad.

MIDDLE EASTERN–SPICED ORZO WITH CHARRED EGGPLANT AND PEPPERS

SERVES 4

1 medium eggplant, about 1 pound, cut into
1-inch cubes

1 large red bell pepper, stemmed, seeded, and cut
into 4 pieces

3 tablespoons extra-virgin olive oil, plus more
for drizzling

Kosher salt and freshly ground black pepper

8 ounces orzo, regular or whole wheat

6 scallions, sliced, white and green parts separated

1 teaspoon ground cumin

½ teaspoon ground allspice

½ teaspoon ground turmeric

¼ teaspoon ground nutmeg

1 tablespoon fresh lemon juice, plus more
as needed

Position an oven rack 6 inches from the heat source and pre-heat the broiler.

Put the eggplant and peppers on a broiler-safe baking sheet, drizzle with olive oil, season with salt and pepper, and toss to combine. Arrange the peppers skin side up; transfer the pan to the oven, and broil, stirring the eggplant halfway through, until blackened all over and softened, 10 to 12 minutes.

Transfer the eggplant to a serving bowl; cool the peppers

briefly, then carefully scrape the charred skins off the peppers with a knife and coarsely chop. Transfer the peppers to the bowl with the eggplant.

Meanwhile, in a large saucepan, cook the orzo in boiling salted water, stirring frequently, until al dente, according to the package instructions. Reserve ½ cup of the cooking water, drain, and transfer to the bowl with the vegetables.

Return the saucepan to the stove over medium heat, and heat until any water in the pan has evaporated; add 3 table-spoons oil to the pan along with the scallion whites, ½ tea-spoon each salt and pepper, cumin, allspice, turmeric, and nutmeg and cook, stirring, until the scallions have softened and the mixture is very fragrant, 3 to 4 minutes. Remove from the heat, stir in the lemon juice, and pour the dress-ing over the orzo and vegetables. Toss, adding splashes of pasta cooking water, until the vegetables and pasta are evenly moistened. Taste and season with additional salt, pepper, and lemon juice.

Stir half of the scallion greens into the mixture and sprin-kle the remainder over the top; serve.

MOROCCAN-SPICED SWEET POTATO WEDGES WITH LEMONY TAHINI SAUCE

SERVES 4

> 4 medium sweet potatoes, about 2½ pounds, peeled and cut into 1-inch wedges
>
> 2 tablespoons extra-virgin olive oil
>
> 1 teaspoon ground cumin
>
> ½ teaspoon ground ginger
>
> ½ teaspoon ground cinnamon
>
> Kosher salt and freshly ground black pepper
>
> ½ cup fat-free plain yogurt
>
> 2 tablespoons fresh lemon juice
>
> 2 tablespoons tahini
>
> 4 scallions, chopped, divided

Preheat the oven to 475°F with a rack positioned in the center. Line a baking sheet with parchment paper.

Put the potato wedges in a large bowl, drizzle the oil over them, and toss to evenly coat. In a small bowl, stir together the cumin, ginger, cinnamon, 1 teaspoon salt, and ½ teaspoon pepper until combined. Sprinkle the spices over the potatoes and toss until evenly coated. Arrange the potatoes cut side down on the baking sheet. Roast until cooked through and deep golden brown, turning once halfway through, 35 to 40 minutes. Cool briefly on the baking sheet.

Meanwhile, in a medium bowl, whisk the yogurt and

lemon together; add the tahini and ½ teaspoon each salt and pepper and mix well. Stir in ¼ cup of the scallions.

Transfer the potatoes to a serving platter and drizzle some of the tahini sauce over them. Sprinkle the rest of the scallions over them, and serve the rest of the sauce at the table.

OVEN-ROASTED MUSHROOM, ARTICHOKE, AND DANDELION GREENS SALAD

SERVES: 4

8 ounces cremini mushrooms, quartered

8 ounces oyster mushrooms, thickly sliced

¼ cup extra-virgin olive oil, divided

Kosher salt and freshly ground black pepper

2 large shallots, thinly sliced into rings

One 12-ounce jar marinated artichoke quarters, drained, plus 2 tablespoons liquid from the jar reserved

1 tablespoon cider or sherry vinegar

1 tablespoon chopped fresh tarragon or 1 teaspoon dried

1 bunch, about 1 pound, dandelion greens, thick stems removed, roughly torn

2 ounces fresh goat cheese or farmer's cheese, crumbled, optional

Preheat the oven to 425°F.

On a large baking sheet, toss the mushrooms with 2 table-spoons of the olive oil until well coated; season well with salt and pepper. Roast in the oven, stirring once halfway through, until the mushrooms release their liquid and begin to brown, about 30 minutes. Remove the baking sheet from the oven, scatter the shallots over the mushrooms, stir well, and return the baking sheet to the oven. Continue roasting until the shallots are softened and just beginning to brown, 6 to 8 minutes; remove from the oven and cool briefly.

Meanwhile, in a large bowl, whisk the remaining olive oil, artichoke liquid, vinegar, tarragon, ½ teaspoon salt, and ¼ teaspoon pepper together until combined. Add the artichokes and ¾ of the mushroom mixture; toss until coated. Add the greens and gently toss until evenly dressed.

Transfer the mixture to a serving platter and scatter the remaining mushrooms and shallots over the top. Garnish with goat cheese crumbles, if using, and serve.

OVEN-ROASTED RADISHES WITH SESAME-MISO BUTTER

SERVES 4

Cooking spray

2 bunches small radishes, such as red, french breakfast, or very small watermelon radish

1 tablespoon grapeseed or sunflower oil

½ cup dairy or vegan butter, softened

2 teaspoons white miso paste

½ teaspoon toasted sesame oil

1 teaspoon toasted white sesame seeds

Coarse salt, such as Maldon or sea salt

Preheat the oven to 400°F. Spray a baking sheet with cooking spray.

Trim the tops of the radishes, leaving 1 inch of the leaf stems attached; rinse well and pat dry. (If the radishes are larger than bite size, halve them lengthwise, being sure to leave some leaf stems attached to each half.) Reserve about 4 of the radish leaves; rinse and pat dry.

Put the radishes on the baking sheet, drizzle the oil over them, and toss well to coat. Roast until crisp-tender and a knife meets little resistance when pierced in the thickest radishes, 20 to 30 minutes. Cool briefly on the baking sheet.

Meanwhile, in a medium bowl, stir together the butter, miso, and sesame oil until smooth and combined. Transfer to a small, wide bowl and set it in the center of a serving platter. Arrange the radishes around the miso butter bowl. Stack the reserved radish leaves and thinly slice into thin ribbons; sprinkle them over the radishes along with the sesame seeds. Serve the radishes with the butter for dipping as a snack or appetizer. Or, if desired, reduce the miso butter amounts by half, mix well, and toss the warm radishes with it until melted, garnishing with the sliced leaves, sesame seeds, and salt as a side dish to a vegetarian meal.

PEARL COUSCOUS WITH SUMMER SQUASH, CHERRY TOMATOES, AND PISTACHIO VINAIGRETTE

SERVES 4

¼ cup extra-virgin olive oil, divided

1 medium sweet onion, chopped

2 cloves garlic, minced

1½ cups pearl couscous

Kosher salt and freshly ground black pepper

2 medium zucchini or yellow squash, about 1 pound, cut into 1-inch chunks

½ cup shelled, chopped pistachios, divided

3 tablespoons cider vinegar

2 teaspoons honey

½ cup fresh parsley leaves

1 pint multicolored cherry tomatoes, halved

Heat 1 tablespoon oil in a large pot over medium-high heat until shimmering. Add the onions and cook, stirring often, until softened, about 5 minutes. Add the garlic and stir for 1 minute. Add the couscous, 1 teaspoon salt, and ½ teaspoon pepper and cook, stirring, until the couscous begins to brown lightly, 3 to 4 minutes.

Stir in the squash and 3 cups water; bring to a boil, stir well, and reduce the heat to maintain a gentle simmer. Cover and cook, stirring occasionally, until the couscous is tender and has absorbed the liquid, about 12 minutes.

Meanwhile, put all but 2 tablespoons of the pistachios in a

blender with the remaining 3 tablespoons oil, vinegar, honey, ½ teaspoon salt, and ¼ teaspoon pepper and blend until smooth. Add the parsley leaves and blend until smooth and bright green. Taste and adjust seasoning if needed.

When the couscous is cooked, stir in the tomatoes, cover, and let stand until softened, about 5 minutes. Stir in the dressing and transfer the couscous to a shallow serving bowl. Garnish with the remaining pistachios and serve.

PAN-SEARED CITRUS CHICKEN

Add a Caribbean splash to your next chicken meal with a bright combination of citrus sections and juices. The trio of grapefruit, orange, and lime join forces to create an exceptional marinade that will make each bit of your chicken burst with sun-filled flavor. Pan searing is an ideal way to cook these breasts because it seals in the juices—and the citrus flavors—and adds a lovely char to the meat's surface.

SERVES 4

> 2 large skinless, boneless chicken breast halves
> (about 1 pound)
> ¼ cup fresh grapefruit juice
> Juice of ½ orange
> Juice of ½ lime
> 2 tablespoons extra-virgin olive oil, divided
> 2 cloves garlic, smashed
> 1 sprig fresh thyme
> Kosher salt and freshly ground black pepper
> 2 cups cooked brown rice (or substitute salad
> greens)

Using a sharp knife, halve the chicken breasts horizontally. Transfer the chicken to a food-safe resealable plastic bag and add the grapefruit, orange, and lime juices; 1 tablespoon of the olive oil; garlic; and thyme. Squeeze the chicken around in the bag with your hands to mix the marinade. Refrigerate for at least 15 minutes and no longer than 30 minutes.

Heat the remaining olive oil in a nonstick skillet over medium heat, swirling to coat the pan. Using tongs, remove the chicken pieces from the bag and shake off the excess marinade. Discard the marinade. Add the chicken to the skillet and season with salt and pepper.

Cook the chicken pieces without moving them until the undersides are golden, about 5 minutes. Flip them, season again with salt and pepper, and cook until the bottoms are golden brown, another 4 to 5 minutes.

Check with an internal-read thermometer—the internal temperature should be at least 165°F. If not, cover and continue cooking until the chicken is cooked through.

Let the chicken rest for a couple of minutes before slicing and serving with the rice.

ROASTED GRAPE, ENDIVE, AND BULGUR SALAD WITH FETA

SERVES 4

2 cups seedless black grapes, halved

⅓ cup extra-virgin olive oil, divided

Kosher salt and freshly ground black pepper

6 scallions, sliced, white and green parts separated

3 tablespoons white balsamic or rice vinegar

2 teaspoons dijon mustard

2 large heads belgian endive, cored, halved, and sliced

2 cups cooked bulgur wheat, cooled

1 head Bibb lettuce, leaves separated

½ cup crumbled feta cheese

Position an oven rack 6 inches from the heat source and preheat the broiler.

Put the grapes on a broiler-safe baking sheet and toss with 1 tablespoon of the oil; season lightly with salt and pepper. Broil, stirring once, until the skins begin to split and the grapes are juicy, 4 to 5 minutes. Remove from the oven and let cool.

Meanwhile, put the scallion whites in a large bowl and pour the vinegar over them; let stand 5 minutes to soften. Add the mustard, ½ teaspoon salt, and ¼ teaspoon black pepper and whisk to dissolve the mustard. While whisking, slowly add the remaining olive oil and mix until combined and thick. Add the grapes and any accumulated juices from the baking sheet, the endive, and half of the scallion greens and toss to coat. Add the bulgur wheat to the bowl, and using a rubber spatula, fold until evenly dressed. Taste and adjust seasoning.

Arrange the lettuce leaves in a single layer on a serving platter. Spoon the bulgur salad over the leaves, evenly scatter the feta over the salad, and sprinkle the remaining scallion greens over the top; serve.

SMOKY ROASTED CAULIFLOWER WEDGES WITH SPICY ALMOND SAUCE

SERVES 4

Cooking spray

1 large head cauliflower, 2 to 2½ pounds, trimmed and cut through the core into 4 wedges

3 tablespoons sunflower or grapeseed oil, divided

Kosher salt and freshly ground black pepper

1 teaspoon smoked paprika

½ teaspoon ground cumin

⅓ cup almond butter

2 tablespoons water

1 to 2 teaspoons hot sauce, such as sriracha or red chili sauce, to taste

2 plum tomatoes, seeded and finely chopped

4 scallions, thinly sliced

Preheat the oven to 425°F. Spray a baking sheet with cooking spray.

Brush the cauliflower wedges all over with 2 tablespoons of the oil. In a small bowl, stir together 1 teaspoon salt, ½ teaspoon black pepper, paprika, and cumin together until combined. Evenly sprinkle half the spice mixture over the cauliflower. Roast in the oven, turning once, until the cauliflower is well browned and a skewer inserted into the center meets little resistance, about 40 minutes. Remove from the oven and let cool briefly.

Meanwhile, in a medium bowl, whisk the almond butter,

water, hot sauce, and remaining spice mixture until combined and smooth; taste and season with salt and pepper. Transfer the cauliflower to a serving platter and drizzle the almond sauce evenly over the wedges. Scatter the tomatoes and scallions over the top and serve.

ORZO SALAD WITH SHRIMP, CUCUMBERS, AND FETA

SERVES 4

3 large strips lemon peel

Juice of 1 lemon, divided

1 clove garlic, smashed

12 whole black peppercorns

12 ounces medium shrimp (41/50), shelled and deveined

1 cup whole-wheat orzo, cooked according to package instructions and rinsed

½ english cucumber, diced

¼ cup chopped fresh dill

2 tablespoons light olive oil

Kosher salt and freshly ground black pepper

4 ounces crumbled feta cheese

In a medium saucepan over medium-high heat, combine 2 cups water with the lemon peel, half the lemon juice, the garlic, and peppercorns, and bring to a boil.

Remove the pan from the heat, stir in the shrimp, and cover. Let stand until the shrimp are cooked through and opaque, about 5 minutes.

Drain the shrimp. Discard the cooking water ingredients and let the shrimp cool to room temperature.

In a mixing bowl, combine the orzo, cucumber, dill, and shrimp, and toss. In another small bowl, combine the remaining lemon juice and olive oil. Whisk until emulsified and season with salt and pepper to taste.

Add the dressing to the orzo and sprinkle with the crumbled cheese. Toss gently until the dressing is absorbed. Serve chilled or at room temperature.

SPAGHETTI SQUASH WITH ALMOND-SAGE PESTO

SERVES 4

> One 2-pound spaghetti squash, halved lengthwise and seeded
>
> ½ cup extra-virgin olive oil, divided, plus more for serving
>
> Kosher salt and freshly ground black pepper
>
> 2 large cloves garlic
>
> ⅓ cup sliced almonds, toasted, plus more for serving
>
> ½ cup loosely packed flat-leaf parsley leaves
>
> ⅓ cup loosely packed fresh sage leaves
>
> ⅓ cup finely grated pecorino romano cheese, plus more for serving

Preheat the oven to 400°F. Place the squash halves in a baking dish and drizzle 2 tablespoons of the oil over the surface; season well with salt and pepper. Place the garlic cloves in the dish, and turn the squash halves over, cut side down, enclosing the garlic underneath. Pour 1 cup water into the dish and cover tightly with aluminum foil. Bake until the squash is tender and the shell begins to collapse, 40 to 45 minutes.

Uncover the squash and carefully turn the halves upright to cool briefly. Transfer the garlic cloves to a food processor along with the almonds. Pulse until the nuts are finely ground and turning into a paste; add the parsley, sage, and cheese and process until smoothly chopped, scraping down the bowl as needed. With the motor running, slowly add the remaining olive oil until combined. Taste and season with salt and pepper.

Using a large fork, scrape the squash halves to remove the long strands and transfer them to a mixing bowl. Add the pesto, and using tongs, toss until well combined. Transfer to a serving bowl and garnish with almonds, pecorino, and a drizzle of olive oil.

SPICY THAI VEGETABLE STIR-FRY

SERVES 4

---

1 small eggplant, about 12 ounces, cut into
1-inch cubes

Kosher salt

¼ cup reduced-sodium soy sauce

2 tablespoons fresh lime juice

1 tablespoon light brown sugar

2 tablespoons sunflower or grapeseed oil

1 small red onion, thinly sliced lengthwise

1 serrano chili, thinly sliced crosswise

1 clove garlic, minced

1 bunch broccolini, about 8 ounces, coarsely
chopped

1 yellow or orange bell pepper, stemmed, seeded,
and thinly sliced

½ cup basil leaves, roughly torn

Steamed rice, for serving

Put the eggplant in a colander, sprinkle with salt, and let stand for 15 minutes. In a small bowl, whisk together the soy sauce, lime juice, and brown sugar until dissolved.

Heat the oil in a wok or large nonstick skillet over medium-high heat until just beginning to smoke. Add the onion and chili and cook, stirring constantly, until softened and beginning to brown, 3 to 4 minutes. Add the garlic and eggplant and stir vigorously until the eggplant is browned on the sides and getting soft, about 5 minutes.

Add the broccolini and peppers and cook, stirring frequently, until the peppers have softened and begin to wilt and the broccolini stems are crisp-tender, 6 to 8 minutes. Pour in the soy mixture and toss until the liquid is simmering, thickens, and glazes the vegetables lightly. Remove from the heat and stir in the basil. Transfer to a shallow bowl and serve hot with rice.

ROASTED BEETS WITH ARUGULA, PISTACHIOS, AND LEMON-SCENTED RICOTTA

SERVES 4

I medium red onion, sliced into 4 thick rounds

4 large beets, scrubbed

I tablespoon extra-virgin olive oil

2 teaspoons balsamic vinegar, divided

Finely grated zest of I lemon

½ cup low-fat ricotta cheese

Kosher salt and freshly ground black pepper

6 cups baby arugula

I teaspoon fresh lemon juice

¼ cup shelled roasted pistachios

Preheat the oven to 400°F.

Lay four 12-inch squares of aluminum foil on a work surface. Set an onion slice on each foil sheet and rest a beet on each onion. Drizzle olive oil and half the vinegar over each and wrap them in the foil.

Place the packets on a baking sheet and roast in the center of the oven until a knife inserted into the beets meets little resistance, 1 to 1¼ hours. Remove from the oven and let stand until cool enough to handle.

Unwrap the packets. Use a paper towel to rub the skin off each beet. Slice the beets into wedges and place them in a bowl. Sprinkle with the remaining vinegar and toss until coated. Separate the roasted onion slices into rings.

In a small bowl, fold the lemon zest into the cheese and season lightly with salt and pepper.

Spread the arugula on a serving platter. Scatter the roasted onion rings over the greens and sprinkle the lemon juice over the top. Season with salt and pepper and toss lightly to dress the greens.

Arrange the beets on top of the greens. Use two spoons to drop dollops of the lemony ricotta all over the salad. Scatter the pistachios over the top and serve.

WHOLE-WHEAT SPAGHETTI WITH SWISS CHARD, WALNUTS, AND PICKLED SHALLOTS

SERVES 4

¼ cup red wine vinegar

1 tablespoon honey

Kosher salt

2 large shallots, thinly sliced

1 bunch green swiss chard, about 1 pound, thick stems removed and chopped, leaves thinly sliced crosswise

1 pound whole-wheat spaghetti

2 tablespoons unsalted butter, optional

½ cup grated pecorino cheese, plus more for serving

½ cup walnuts, toasted and coarsely chopped, divided

Freshly ground black pepper

In a medium bowl, stir the vinegar, honey, and ½ teaspoon salt together until combined; add the shallots and toss to submerge them. Let stand for 10 minutes while you cook the pasta.

Bring 2 quarts of water to a boil; add 1 tablespoon salt, the chard stems, and pasta, and cook, stirring frequently, until al dente, according to the package instructions. Remove 1½ cups of the cooking water; drain the pasta and stems and reserve in the colander.

Pour 1 cup of the cooking water into the pasta pot and bring to a vigorous simmer over medium-high heat. Add the sliced chard and cook, tossing, until wilted, 2 to 3 minutes. Add the pasta and stems and cook, tossing, until the liquid is bubbling. Add the butter and cheese and toss until melted and smooth, adding more cooking water as needed to make a silky sauce. Add half the walnuts and toss; taste and season with salt and pepper.

Transfer the pasta to a serving platter and garnish with additional cheese. Drain the excess liquid from the shallots and scatter them over the top of the spaghetti along with the remaining walnuts; serve.

10

PLANT
POWER
SNACKS

Below you will find a list of snacks that you might choose from on the Plant Power plan. This is not meant to be a comprehensive list, as the snack options are virtually limitless. But this is a good starting point for you to get your snack groove on. The snack list is conveniently separated into plant-based and animal-based to facilitate your search. The vast majority of these snacks are 150 calories or less. Stick to the portion size as closely as possible, but feel free to get creative by mixing and matching some of the ingredients. Experiment and have fun!

PLANT-BASED FOODS (PBF)

- Small baked potato topped with salsa
- ¾ cup roasted cauliflower slices with a pinch of sea salt
- ½ large cucumber, cut in sticks or coins, dipped in 2 tablespoons hummus
- 1 cup Cheerios

- 2 fresh pineapple rings, each ¼ inch thick, grilled or sautéed
- 2 stalks celery and 2 tablespoons organic peanut butter
- 3 medium breadsticks with 2 tablespoons hummus
- 1½ cups fresh fruit salad
- ⅓ cup unsweetened applesauce and ½ cup dry cereal
- ¾ cup roasted chickpeas
- 1 medium corn on the cob with seasoning
- 3 hummus-and-veggie roll-ups
- ¾ cup roasted almonds and 5 dried cherries
- 3 tablespoons tomato dip (1 large tomato, ½ teaspoon minced garlic, 2 tablespoons olive oil, and 15 almonds blended in a food processor until smooth) and 4 pita wedges
- ¾ cup pico de gallo and 5 tortilla chips
- Homemade sweet potato chips: Thinly slice 2 sweet potatoes and place in a bowl with 2 tablespoons olive oil and sea salt to taste. Place on an aluminum foil–lined baking sheet and bake in a 375-degree oven for 25 to 30 minutes until desired crispness. (Eat 1 cup of chips and save the rest for later.)
- ½ cup nut-free trail mix with no added sugar
- 4 dried apricots with 15 dry-roasted almonds
- Organic nut or protein bar (150 calories or less)
- 11 blue-corn tortilla chips
- 1 medium mango
- 25 frozen red seedless grapes
- 5 tortilla chips and ⅓ cup guacamole
- 1 large apple, sliced, sprinkled with cinnamon
- 6 dried figs

- 20 grapes with 15 peanuts
- Watermelon salad: 1 cup raw spinach with ⅔ cup diced watermelon, sprinkled with 1 tablespoon balsamic vinegar
- 1 cup lettuce drizzled with 2 tablespoons fat-free dressing
- 3 oven-baked potato wedges
- 3 crackers lightly spread with organic peanut butter
- 2 graham cracker squares and 2 teaspoons nut butter, sprinkled with cinnamon
- 10 chocolate-covered almonds
- 16 cashews
- 2 medium-size nectarines
- ½ cup mini pretzels and 1 teaspoon honey mustard
- ½ medium avocado sprinkled with a little squeeze of lime juice and sea salt
- 20 raw almonds
- 3 cups air-popped popcorn
- 1½ cups puffed rice
- 2 tablespoons refried bean dip (made without lard) and 5 tortilla chips
- Black bean salsa over 3 roasted eggplant slices
- 16 saltines
- ½ cup avocado topped with diced tomatoes and a pinch of pepper
- 2 medium kiwis, sliced
- 3 fresh figs
- 25 roasted peanuts
- 2 tablespoons shelled sunflower seeds
- 1 cup radishes, sliced or chopped, drizzled with balsamic vinaigrette

- 17 pecan halves
- 1 cup sliced zucchini (roasted if you desire) seasoned with salt to taste
- Kale chips: ⅔ cup raw kale baked with 1 teaspoon olive oil at 400 degrees until crisp
- ¼ cup loosely packed raisins
- 1 pomegranate
- 2 frozen fruit bars (no sugar added)
- ½ cup quinoa or brown rice
- 2 cups watermelon chunks
- ½ small apple, sliced with 2 teaspoons nut butter
- White bean salad: ½ cup white beans, squeeze of lemon juice, ¼ cup diced tomatoes, 4 cucumber slices
- 10 baby carrots dipped in 2 tablespoons light salad dressing
- 2 small peaches
- 1 large raw carrot
- 1 cup mixed berries (strawberries, blueberries, blackberries, raspberries)
- Crispy asparagus: Wash and trim 8 asparagus spears. In a bowl, mix 1½ tablespoons shelled sunflower seeds, ½ teaspoon garlic powder, juice of ½ lemon, ¼ cup whole-wheat bread crumbs, a pinch of ground pepper, and a pinch of paprika. Lay the spears on a baking sheet and evenly cover each spear with the bread crumb mixture. Bake in a preheated oven at 350 degrees for 20 to 30 minutes until crispy.
- 6 pieces of veggie sushi rolls
- ½ cup small pretzels and 2 tablespoons hummus
- ½ cup cooked organic instant oatmeal with berries

- 20 organic seaweed snacks
- 1 baked tofu bar
- 2 scoops of sorbet
- ½ cup roasted lupini beans
- ¼ cup cashews with ¼ cup dried cranberries
- 1 cup baked apple chips
- Plant-based crackers (amount equal to 150 calories or less)
- 1 fruit bar
- 5 pitted dates stuffed with 5 whole almonds
- 40 shelled pistachios
- ¾ cup melon cubes
- 1 stalk celery cut into sections and 2 tablespoons nut butter
- 3 pineapple rings in natural juices, no sugar added
- 10 baby carrots dipped in 2 tablespoons light salad dressing
- 3 to 4 tablespoons dried cherries
- 8 to 10 slices cucumber and 2 tablespoons hummus
- Watermelon and honeydew melon balls (8 total)
- 1 slice 100 percent whole-wheat bread or 1 whole-grain pita pocket, cut into quarters, with 2 tablespoons hummus
- 2 cups air-popped popcorn drizzled with a rosemary-lemon combo made from combining and heating 2 teaspoons olive oil, 2 teaspoons minced rosemary, ¼ teaspoon grated lemon zest, and a pinch of sea salt
- Homemade trail mix: Combine 7 roasted almonds, 2 tablespoons dried cranberries, 5 mini pretzel twists, and 1 tablespoon shelled sunflower seeds.
- Sweet walnut oatmeal (½ cup cooked steel-cut oats topped with 1 tablespoon chopped walnuts and drizzled with 1 teaspoon organic honey or 100 percent maple syrup)

- ½ cup sweet potato chips
- ¾ cup cooked carrots
- 4 dried apricots with 1 tablespoon dried cherries
- Small kale salad (1 cup kale leaves topped with ½ cup roasted chickpeas drizzled with tahini dressing)
- 15 frozen banana slices (usually 1 large banana)
- ½ large grapefruit sprinkled with ½ teaspoon sugar, broiled if desired
- Small green garden salad (greens, tomatoes, olives, shredded carrots)
- 10 walnut halves and 1 sliced kiwi
- Baby burrito: Spread 2 tablespoons bean dip on a 6-inch corn tortilla and top with 2 tablespoons salsa.
- 1 cup grapes with 10 almonds
- ¾ cup roasted black beans
- 1 cup sugar snap peas with 3 tablespoons hummus
- ¾ cup steamed edamame, seasoned and salted to taste
- ½ cup pretzels and 1 teaspoon honey mustard
- Kale bruschetta: Toast 1 slice 100 percent whole-grain or 100 percent whole-wheat bread, top with cooked kale leaves and halved grape tomatoes, salt and pepper to taste, and drizzle with balsamic vinaigrette.
- Small baked potato (white or sweet) topped with 2 tablespoons hummus
- Dehydrated cinnamon apples: Thinly slice 3 medium apples. Sprinkle with cinnamon. Spread evenly on parchment paper in a baking dish. Place in a 170-degree oven for 5 to 6 hours, turning the slices every hour until browned and crispy. (Eat 1 apple's worth of slices as a snack and save the other two for later.)

- ½ red bell pepper, sliced, drizzled with balsamic vinaigrette and seasoned with salt and pepper
- Mediterranean salad: Dice 1 tomato, 1 small cucumber, and ¼ red onion. Drizzle with balsamic vinaigrette.
- Black bean salsa over 3 roasted eggplant slices
- ¼ red bell pepper, sliced, ¼ cup thin carrot slices, ¼ cup guacamole
- 1 cup miso soup
- 1 tablespoon peanuts and 2 tablespoons dried cranberries
- 50 Goldfish crackers
- ½ cup kale chips
- 3 tablespoons roasted pumpkin seeds
- 1 large apple, orange, or banana
- 4 almond butter–stuffed dates
- ½ cup black beans topped with 2 tablespoons guacamole
- 6 dates
- 1½ cups vegan chili topped with avocado slices
- ½ cup unsweetened applesauce mixed with 10 pecan halves
- ¼ cup low-fat granola
- 2 tablespoons hummus spread on 4 crackers
- 5 baby carrots and 3 tablespoons hummus
- 2 cups grilled or roasted broccoli florets
- 25 cherries
- 1 rice cake with 1 tablespoon guacamole
- 2 dill pickle spears
- ½ cup wasabi peas
- ½ cup raw or cooked vegetables

- 12 baked tortilla chips and ½ cup salsa
- 1 cup grape tomatoes, halved and sprinkled with sea salt
- ½ sheet matzo
- 1 baked sweet potato with 1 teaspoon butter
- ¼ avocado, smashed, on a whole-grain cracker, sprinkled with balsamic vinegar and sea salt
- 3 tablespoons roasted unsalted soy nuts
- 4 saltine jelly sandwiches: sugar-free jelly between 2 saltine crackers; 8 crackers in all
- 1 fruit breakfast bar (150 calories or less)
- 1 healthy granola bar (150 calories or less)
- 1 medium tomato, sliced, with a pinch of salt
- Black bean salsa over 3 roasted eggplant slices
- 1 cup strawberries
- 6 dried apricots
- 1 cup grape tomatoes
- 10 black olives
- 1 vegan blueberry muffin and 1 serving of fruit
- 1 cup dairy-free chia seed pudding
- Fresh fruit platter with 3 to 4 servings of fruit

ANIMAL-BASED FOODS (ABF)

- 1 cup blueberries with a dollop of whipped cream
- Tomato-mozzarella salad: Cube 1 ounce fresh mozzarella and combine in a small bowl with 11 halved cherry tomatoes and 2 teaspoons chopped fresh basil, then drizzle with 1 tablespoon balsamic vinaigrette.

- 1 small scoop low-fat frozen yogurt
- Greek tomatoes: Chop 1 medium tomato and mix with 1 tablespoon feta cheese and a squeeze of lemon juice; add a sprinkle of oregano if desired.
- Hot quesadilla: Spray 1 side of a corn tortilla with cooking spray, then place in a skillet over medium heat. Top with ¼ cup Mexican cheese blend, fold in half, and cook for a couple of minutes on each side until the cheese melts and the tortilla is slightly crisp. Serve with 2 tablespoons pico de gallo or salsa if desired.
- Spicy black beans: ¼ cup black beans with 1 tablespoon salsa and 1 tablespoon fat-free plain Greek yogurt
- ½ cup canned crab
- 3 ounces cooked fresh crab
- 3 dried apricots stuffed with 1 tablespoon crumbled blue cheese
- Stuffed tomatoes: 10 halved grape tomatoes stuffed with a mixture of ¼ cup low-fat ricotta cheese, 1 tablespoon diced black olives, and a pinch each of pepper and sea salt
- 4 cooked large sea scallops
- ½ cup low-fat cottage cheese with ¼ cup fresh pineapple slices
- 1 cup fresh red raspberries topped with ½ cup low-fat yogurt
- 1 medium red bell pepper, sliced, with 2 tablespoons soft goat cheese
- 5 cucumber slices topped with ⅓ cup cottage cheese and sprinkled with salt and pepper

- 1 slice swiss cheese and 8 olives
- 2 cups air-popped popcorn with 1 teaspoon butter
- 2 ounces smoked salmon (no added sugar)
- ½ cup pudding of your choice
- 3 celery sticks stuffed with cottage cheese (each stick should be 5 inches long)
- 1 portobello mushroom stuffed with roasted veggies and 1 teaspoon shredded low-fat cheese
- 8 small shrimp and 2 tablespoons cocktail sauce
- 1 cup chicken noodle soup
- ½ cup light natural vanilla ice cream or sorbet
- 10 cooked mussels
- Open-faced turkey swiss melt: On half of a whole-wheat english muffin, place ¾ ounce low-sodium deli turkey and 1 thin slice swiss cheese. Melt and serve.
- 4 turkey slices and 1 medium apple, sliced
- 1 fat-free mozzarella cheese stick with ½ medium apple, sliced
- 2 hard-boiled eggs with a pinch of salt and pepper
- Chocolate-dipped pretzels: Melt 1 tablespoon semisweet chocolate morsels in a microwave. Dip 3 honey pretzel sticks in the chocolate. Put the pretzels in the freezer until the chocolate sets.
- 1 ounce cheddar cheese with 5 radishes
- Cucumber sandwich: ½ english muffin topped with 2 tablespoons cottage cheese and 3 slices cucumber
- 1 hard-boiled egg and ½ cup sugar snap peas
- 6 cucumber, cherry tomato, and mozzarella ball skewers
- 2 ounces beef or turkey jerky

- 4 chocolate chip cookies, each a little larger than the size of a poker chip
- Turkey-wrapped avocado: ¼ avocado sliced and wrapped in 3 ounces low-sodium deli turkey meat
- ½ cucumber (seeded) stuffed with 1 thin slice lean turkey and mustard or fat-free mayonnaise
- 10 baby carrots with ½ cup cottage cheese that's been mixed with ½ tablespoon pesto sauce
- Yogurt-dipped strawberries: Dip a cup of whole strawberries in ½ cup low-fat vanilla Greek yogurt, place on a baking sheet, and freeze.
- 1 cup 2 percent ultra-filtered chocolate milk
- Peanut butter chocolate square: 0.4-ounce chocolate square topped with 2 teaspoons creamy organic peanut butter
- ½ cup diced cantaloupe topped with ½ cup low-fat cottage cheese
- 3 ounces water-packed tuna, drained and seasoned to taste
- 4 meat-based pot stickers dipped in 2 teaspoons reduced-sodium soy sauce
- 2 ounces lean roast beef
- 8-ounce container Greek yogurt
- ½ cup cottage cheese and almond butter
- 1 hard-boiled egg with everything bagel seasoning
- 1 small pear sliced and spread with 1 tablespoon almond butter
- ¼ cup shredded chicken breast served on 5 whole-wheat crackers and topped with 2 tablespoons low-fat shredded cheese and salsa

- 1 whole-grain waffle topped with 2 tablespoons low-fat or fat-free plain yogurt and ½ cup berries
- 1 small apple, sliced and dipped into ½ cup low-fat cottage cheese and sprinkled with cinnamon
- 4 ounces chicken breast wrapped in lettuce and topped with dill mustard
- 7 olives stuffed with 1 tablespoon blue cheese
- 1 can water-packed tuna, drained and seasoned to taste
- 6 oysters
- 1 small chocolate pudding
- Honey-ricotta rice cake: Spread 3 tablespoons ricotta cheese over 1 brown rice cake, then drizzle with 2 teaspoons honey.
- Chocolate graham cracker: Cover 2 graham cracker squares with 2 teaspoons chocolate hazelnut spread and form a sandwich.
- 1 sweet apple, such as Golden Delicious or Fuji, with reduced-fat sharp cheddar cheese stick or ¾-ounce slice
- 1 cup steamed vegetables with 1 ounce melted reduced-fat cheese
- 1 chopped hard-cooked egg mixed with 2 teaspoons light mayo served on cucumber slices and 5 whole-wheat crackers
- Egg and hot sauce sandwich: 1 whole-grain english muffin topped with ½ cup cooked egg whites and drizzled with hot sauce
- 2 slices 100 percent whole-grain or 100 percent whole-wheat toast spread with 2 tablespoons almond butter

- ½ cup low-fat or fat-free plain Greek yogurt with a dash of cinnamon and 1 teaspoon honey
- 6 large clams
- Turkey roll-ups: 4 slices smoked turkey rolled up and dipped in 2 teaspoons honey mustard

INDEX

INDEX